METHADONE:
BAD BOY
of Drug Treatment

D0110078

METHADONE:
BAD BOY
of Drug Treatment
What Works & What Doesn't

REBECCA JANES, LMHC, LADC

Outskirts Press, Inc.
Denver, Colorado

Methadone: Bad Boy of Drug Treatment
What Works & What Doesn't
All Rights Reserved.
Copyright © 2010 Rebecca Janes, LMHC, LADC
v2.0

Outskirts Press, Inc.
http://www.outskirtspress.com

ISBN: 978-1-4327-5074-9

Outskirts Press and the "OP" logo are trademarks belonging to Outskirts Press, Inc.

PRINTED IN THE UNITED STATES OF AMERICA

"Most addicts use drugs to hide from overwhelming feelings. They don't know any healthier ways to tolerate them. Recovery is about looking inside and trying to change. Methadone acts as a safe platform from which you can learn to handle the addiction from the inside out."-

N.M., a methadone client

This book is dedicated to the many good souls I've met on the clinic- among them are some who have died too soon:

Priscilla, George, Celeste, John

Contents

Introduction.. 1

CHAPTER ONE
Mistaken Beliefs of the General Public 5
1. "Methadone junkies"- aren't they just getting high at the taxpayers' expense?...5
2. "How about that new alternative buprenorphine/ Suboxone: wasn't that supposed to take the place of methadone?" 14
3. "Methadone doesn't work--Nobody ever gets off the clinic." 18
4. "The clinic just wants to keep clients there for the money.".. 23
5. Heroin is worse than pills." 25
6. "Heroin is worse than cocaine." 29
7. "Heroin is worse than alcohol." 34
8. "People on methadone aren't 'clean.' " 35
9. "I hear people are dying from methadone over-dose.".. 36
10. "People on methadone don't need pain medication, since methadone is a pain medicine.".................... 38

CHAPTER TWO
Misinformation Addicts tell each Other 41
1. "Methadone is 'liquid handcuffs.'"........................... 41
2. "It eats your bones." 45
3. "It rots your teeth.".. 46
4. "You'll get fat.".. 47
5. "Methadone makes you crave sweets." 49
6. "Methadone makes you crave cocaine.".................. 50
7. "It's harder to kick than dope." 51
8. "I've heard 'they' can 'put you out' and filter your blood in one day to get off of methadone (or opiates)." 54

9. "I got on the clinic for opiates- it's none of their business if I do cocaine, alcohol or pot." 56

10. "I just need the methadone, I don't need counseling," or -"Just give me my dose." 58

11. "I can't stand groups; everybody just tells 'war stories.'." 59

12. "My counselor never even used drugs- how can he/she help an addict?" 60

CHAPTER THREE

What Doesn't Work in Methadone Treatment 61

1. shaming 61

2. When well intentioned people try to push clients to get off the clinic... 63

3. Time limits on treatment. 65

4. Limits on dose. 66

5. Dosing without counseling. 67

6. Treating the addiction without treating the psychiatric problem. 68

7. Allowing other addictions to replace the opiates (including legally prescribed drugs) 76

8. Inconsistency and too much "leeway" 77

9. "A higher level of care": the little white lie 78

CHAPTER FOUR

What Works in Methadone Treatment 81

1. Respect: Using new ideas that work- 81

2. Getting people into treatment more quickly 84

3. Supervised, reliable drug tests 86

4. Clear rules, with plenty of second chances 87

5. Strong rewards for any progress 89

6. On-site psychiatric help 91

7. Inpatient detox for cocaine, more effective long term residential programs, and "Safe Houses" 92

8. Group process... 93
9. Encouraging clients who are stable to slowly detox-- without deadlines-... 95
10. Help with reintegrating into the community 97
11. Opportunities and incentives to get off disability and earn a decent wage 98

CHAPTER FIVE
Some Hard Decisions 101
1. "the Reality Principle".............................. 101
2. Disability/methadone- A formula for depression and obesity... 101
3. Rethinking Pain treatment- 103
4. Rethinking Anxiety treatment- 106
5. More comprehensive (and realistic) treatment for cocaine.. 109
6. The rights of the unborn child vs. the rights of the addicted mother 109
7. Better support for dealing with Domestic Violence issues 112

CHAPTER SIX
The Future of Opiate Treatment-..115

Bibliography 119

Methadone:

Bad Boy of Drug Treatment

What works, and what doesn't

Introduction

⤜᷃᷁᷄⤛

*Methadone is a medicine that is used to help people who have become physically dependent on opiates. These people may have been using illegal opiates (heroin, or prescription pain killers used illegally), or may have been on opiates legally for medical conditions but are having difficulty withdrawing from them. It is sometimes used to treat chronic pain. The good part is that methadone is legal, and very effective at stopping the extreme "flu-like" symptoms of physical withdrawal, and will make it hard for a person to get "high" on other opiates. The bad part is that the person is then physically dependent on the methadone, which is actually harder to get off of than the heroin (but not impossible).

Methadone treatment is far from perfect, and it is not the only effective treatment for opiate dependence. In fact, it is one of the most despised treatment options. However, despite its reputation, the U.S. government considers it to be one of the most effective treatments available (*NIDA*), and, for some clients, it is the only one that helps.

Methadone is a tool in drug abuse treatment. As with any tool, it can be used or it can be abused.

METHADONE: BAD BOY OF DRUG TREATMENT

Before working in the substance abuse field, I thought it seemed just too convenient that all the plots on crime shows and movies led back to drugs. Now, after fourteen years working as a counselor at a methadone clinic, it seems all too true. The scale of harm done by illicit drugs to our culture, our economy, and to our poorest citizens is overwhelming. Working with the clients, as the individuals they are, keeps the work worth doing. Meanwhile, our nation has some very big, politically sensitive, and uncomfortable decisions to make.

Few people realize how much impact the failure of our "war on drugs" has had on our Social Security/disability and healthcare/Medicare programs. Illicit drugs and alcohol abuse are two of the biggest factors connected to homelessness and disability in this nation; another is chronic mental illness. More often than not, the substance abuse and chronic mental illness are inseparable. To improve our drug programs we need to improve our treatment of mental illness. To curb the impact of illicit drugs we, as a culture, need to take more responsibility for our physical health, and change our expectations of pain control.

For those readers who are suffering from addiction, this book is written in the hope that you will find effective treatment, and make good use of it.

For those who are looking for help for a loved one, you are not alone. There are few families who are not haunted by addiction. Most families hide the problem, either blaming themselves or the addict. It is time to talk about what will make all our good intentions actually help. We need to find the balance that avoids the extremes of either enabling, or condemning and giving up on the addicted person.

INTRODUCTION

As a nation, we need to look at our drug treatment programs and, instead of continuing to do what is not working or is hardly working, start doing what will solve the larger problems.

After years of seeing what works and what doesn't in methadone treatment, this book offers a personal opinion of how some of the popular and persistent beliefs about methadone, and drug treatment in general, effect some of those larger problems.

Many of the accusations and misunderstandings about methadone treatment contain an element of truth, but they are only partly true, or arc problems that can be fixed. The idea that they comprise the whole truth can sabotage the best hope for a very vulnerable population. Opiate addiction is a complex problem and devastating to anyone it touches, and we need every tool possible to fight it.

Methadone is one tool in recovery from opiate dependence. We can use it effectively, or use it clumsily and harmfully. For many clients it has already been a lifesaver. It could help many more with some understanding, and well- thought-out programs that have community support.

CHAPTER ONE

Mistaken Beliefs
of the General Public

1. *"Methadone junkies"- aren't they just getting high at the taxpayers' expense?*

Telling people that my job is at a methadone clinic almost always brings the same response: "Aren't they just getting high at taxpayers' expense?"

This actually represents two assumptions: (A) that people are high when they are on methadone and (B) that there is an alternate or cheaper way to take care of the drug problem other than funding by the government.

A *"They're just getting high"*

For non-informed readers, let me explain about the dose level. As with many drugs such as Depakote, lithium, or Coumadin, the level of medicine in the blood needs to be "just right"---not too high, and not too low. If the blood level is too high it will be toxic; if it is too low it will be ineffective. This appropriate range is the "therapeutic level," meaning the medicine is doing what it is supposed to do.

When the methadone is within this therapeutic range, clients do not feel the symptoms of withdrawal. In other words, they feel "normal." If the blood level falls below that, they start feeling the discomfort of withdrawal. If it is above the therapeutic level, it becomes toxic. This toxic effect, which will happen with nearly any medicine at some level, is what produces the drowsiness, the "nod" of feeling high.

When clients first get on methadone, they may feel some drowsiness as they adjust to their dosage. This should subside after a few days.

Certain medications, as well as stress, can change the clients' need for methadone. When clients say they are still feeling discomfort and want to increase their dosage, they will be checked for signs of withdrawal by a nurse, and have the change order signed off by a doctor before the dose is increased. Before the dose is put unusually high, the clients' methadone blood level should be checked. This costs extra and, of course, depends on sufficient funds to give proper treatment. How high a dose is too high? There is no one-size-fits-all answer. This will be discussed in more detail later.

Are there clients who "play" with their dose in an attempt to get this feeling of being "high"? Of course. This is a population that has difficulty facing life without that escape. So, some clients might try to get their dose increased in order to get "high" for a couple of days before their bodies adjust.

So, why is there a stereotype of the methadone client nodding out and drooling in the waiting room? My guess is that most of the clients fitting that description are supplementing their dose with scripts, or with illicit drugs, or both. The majority of these "supplements" fall in the category of benzodiazepines, but some are non-narcotic. We'll discuss this more extensively later.

B. "At taxpayers' expense"

The second part of the question is whether there is a cheaper way to "clean up" the drug problem, or a way to avoid having our taxes pay for it.

As for other sources of money, to my knowledge there has never been a telethon or a bake sale for drug treatment. (I have recently heard of one exception: A mother has been running marathons to raise awareness and money for drug treatment after getting help for her step daughter.)

Every few years someone in our Massachusetts State Legislature will try to cut the funding for methadone. That earlier reference to "methadone junkies" was a quote from one of these legislators. If the funding did get cut, a crime wave would likely hit that would send the lawmakers scrambling back to the drawing board.

My job is in the small New England city of New Bedford, Massachusetts. With a population of 100,000, there are two methadone clinics, each with several hundred clients. Admittedly, some of those clients still commit crimes frequently, but there are many others who are working in the community. There are probably a lot more of these than the general public imagines. And the methadone allows them to "normalize" their lives, keeping their families intact, and their health in order, while controlling symptoms of withdrawal.

And there are many more methadone clients who, though temporarily unable to work, are slowly trying to calm the chaos of their past: paying off court fines, getting their driver's licenses back, getting their kids out of foster care,

getting overdue psychiatric and medical treatment.....
Hopefully, they are also learning more healthy ways to
deal with those uncomfortable emotions and situations
that life presents.

Picture what would happen if these people were suddenly
thrown into serious withdrawal all at once. Opiate-addicted
individuals generally have a terrible fear of withdrawal
symptoms. When looking for a description of how withdrawal feels, I asked some clients whether it is like "a
terrible case of the flu." They all reacted at once: *"It's so
much worse because you're so terrified at the same time.
I would take the flu ten times over to avoid withdrawal."*

There may be a few individuals who would try not to resort
to stealing for the drugs necessary to ease their physical
symptoms, but not many. Their symptoms would last over
a month, and, by then their lives would be in chaos again.
Of course, in reality, since most would have reverted to using street drugs, their symptoms would last until they were
able to get into treatment again (or until they were incar-
cerated or dead).

This is not a problem that will resolve itself without
intervention.

Fortunately, this scenario is unlikely to happen. The clinics depend heavily on federal, not just state support, and
the federal government believes more in methadone than
many local officials, and would not support the state's cutting off these funds.

Even those taxpayers who have no sympathy for the addict
should look at the bottom line of how much we pay for not

providing effective treatment.

So how else can we deal with the drug problem?

Why don't we let them kill themselves off?

This has been made as a "joking" suggestion for dealing with the problem. As with any sarcastic remark, (known in psychotherapy as a particularly nasty form of passive- aggressive behavior), people who make this suggestion may have an unrealistic idea of who they are including.

This is not only about those nameless "dark alley junkies." Think about the many elderly people who are being treated for chronic pain and have become dependent. And how about our children? Remember the idea that, "But for the grace of God, go I (or my child)?" This is about some of our best and brightest. It includes those young people getting addicted to their grandmother's pain meds.

The generation now getting hooked on pills will come to the place where their habit is too expensive to manage. Illicit pills are much more expensive than heroin. Some friend, lover, or dealer will tell them so, and they will inevitably go down that dark alley if they do not get into effective treatment first.

We treasure our free society where people are allowed to live as they choose. We can't tell people not to eat junk food when they are killing themselves by overeating. We can't forbid cigarettes to emphysema patients, or liquor to people with cirrhosis. Our taxes take care of those who are disabled by their unhealthy eating, smoking, and drinking habits.

Is one addiction more "acceptable" than the other? Of course. Some addictions are obviously more politically or socially "correct" in our culture. Some people look the other way at pot, cocaine, certainly nicotine, and, of course, alcohol---not to mention gambling, junk food, and shopping, but are horrified by the specter of heroin. We need to move away from moral judgments of one addiction over another.

Recovery and relapse prevention principles and skills are basically the same. We all have to learn how to cope with uncomfortable emotions and overwhelming situations, our own mortality, and the general unfairness of life. Those of us who have been lucky enough to have healthy coping mechanisms modeled for us by a loving family, or teachers, or mentors, are less likely to turn to, or become entangled in, the unhealthy addictions that others fall into.

> ** To the family members reading this, who have done the best they could, there are other contributing factors that can and do counteract your best efforts. This is not to imply blame.*

If addicts overdose, why do we have to pay to save them?

Whether the overdose is intentional or not, our society is still acting on the principle that suicide is illegal. Many addicts die from overdose. Many survive to use again. And many have serious medical problems, some caused by drug use and some not.

Currently more methadone clients die of cigarette addiction than illegal drugs.

We pay for people who do all kinds of crazy things and end up in trouble. Our tradition of Christian morality dictates, "Don't judge if you don't want to be judged," and all major religions teach us to "treat others the way you want them to treat you." If we support the belief that we are a "moral society," then we have to try to help people in trouble, whether they fall down a well or fall into addiction, and we must leave the judging to God, "a higher power," "karma," or whoever or whatever we believe is in charge.

So, should we just put all the junkies in jail?

Shall we imprison alcoholics? No, because, of course, they can obtain their "drug of choice" legally. Using heroin and other opiates not prescribed to that person is already against the law. So should we keep them in jail longer to clean up our cities? Remember Scrooge's line, "Are there no prisons? Are there no poorhouses?"

Apart from the moral niceties, this doesn't even work out on a practical level. The cost of keeping one person in jail for a year is over $20,000 and that person in a methadone clinic costs about $8,000 a year. Some estimates are even more dramatic:

> *"The cost of addictions treatment is 15 times less than the cost of incarcerating a person for a drug related crime."*
>
> *PLNDP and Join Together*

We already pay a lot for drug abusers who are not in treatment, and we pay a lot for ineffective treatment.

Our taxes pay for their ambulance rides, their medical care, their disabilities caused by the physical damage of drug abuse. We pay the Department of Social Services to monitor their children or take custody, and then we pay for foster care. We pay for the police work, the court and probation systems; we pay for the high insurance for protecting property and businesses. We pay for "revolving door" detoxes.

Methadone is acknowledged by our federal government to be the most effective, and the most cost effective treatment we have at this time for people who have tried detox and failed repeatedly to control opiate addiction. *(NIDA)*

Why aren't inpatient detoxes enough?

Inpatient detoxes are an important part of drug treatment. When the client is physically destroying him- or herself and has lost any hope of getting the drug use under control, it is the only appropriate treatment. For some people, who are motivated, and have strong social and family support, a detox can work. The problem comes when a person is released from a detox to the same unhealthy social surroundings that they were in before.

Most of my clients have tried inpatient detoxes time after time before getting on methadone. They report often relapsing before they reach home. Sometimes, they have already called their drug connection before they leave.

Many clients remember when an inpatient detox would last 30 days. Now insurance dictates that they usually can stay only five days, since the worst physical withdrawal symptoms from opiates are over by then.

This does not leave time for the person to deal with the social, financial, and physical devastation that they have put themselves through. They still believe that the only way they can feel better when they are angry, or anxious, or depressed, is to get high.

Inpatient detoxes are too brief to treat most opiate addiction.

Think of the person addicted to cigarettes who has surgery and stays in the hospital for two weeks without being able to smoke cigarettes. He or she thinks of nothing else but getting that first cigarette on the way home. They know they shouldn't smoke. The physical withdrawal is over. Their doctors have told them it will kill them. Their families plead with them to stop. But, with few exceptions, they smoke. This happens even though the physical withdrawal symptoms are gone. The emotional and psychiatric problems that have gotten that person addicted in the first place have not changed. If these are not treated, relapse is almost inevitable. They still believe that the only way to keep themselves from getting overwhelmed by feeling angry, or anxious, or depressed, is to have a cigarette. (Or heroin, if that has been their coping mechanism) .

Methadone is acknowledged by the United States federal government to be the most effective, and the most cost effective treatment we have at this time for people who have tried detox and failed repeatedly to control opiate addiction.

So the question is not how to stop spending on drug treatment, but how to make our tax dollars do what we want them to do, as efficiently as possible.

Doesn't it make sense to get as many people into treatment as soon as possible, and to do our best to make that treatment work?

2. *"How about that new alternative buprenorphine/Suboxone: wasn't that supposed to take the place of methadone?"*

Buprenorphine (Suboxone/Suboxyl) was billed as the "Great New Hope" for opiate addiction. We wouldn't need the daily methadone dosing and the unwieldy expensive structure of a methadone clinic. Doctors can prescribe a month of pills at a time, and are, of course, supposed to track each client so they get drug screens and regular counseling. It is less addictive, and it is easier to detox from it. As a matter of fact, the way the protocol was first written, treatment was supposed to last only 90 days. Problem solved. Case closed.

Suboxone is a great addition to opiate addiction treatment, and for some clients it is an excellent choice. When the government set up the guidelines for this new drug treatment they tried to make sure it would not become a street drug.

Our lawmakers put in special safeguards to make this work:

Only certain doctors are approved to dispense buprenorphine. They attend an eight-hour training to become certified (or do it online).

At first doctors were limited to prescribing this drug to only 30 clients at a time. This has been raised to 100, on the assumption that doctors have the tracking system in place by now.

To assure the Suboxone would not be abused, the wafers are mixed with Naloxone/Narcan.

This is the drug used to bring someone out of an overdose. It "knocks" the person out of the "high". This meant that the prescription would not be used with other opiates since the other opiates "high" would not be felt.

Unfortunately, things didn't go as planned-

Our lawmakers underestimated the ingenuity of the drug culture. Suboxone is now a very popular street drug, and widely available. I have spoken with clients who say they have used it to get high. It is used for sniffing, for shooting up, as well as to help someone get *"straight"* (not feel the withdrawal symptoms) until they can get their drug of choice.

As one of my clients confided, "As far as Suboxone goes, the wafer is usually sold in quarters: $2.50 a quarter. Junkies usually buy them like that, because if they had $10 they'd buy dope." Others said it can be up to $20 or $25 a wafer.

Another problem with Suboxone treatment: it is easy to take "vacations" from it. The Naloxone is gone from the system quickly, so the client can choose to go get high after one to three days, depending on the dose. This also means that the client then has extra wafers, which have street value. *Now he has supplemental income, often courtesy of his insurance.*

Another way clients can have a supply to sell is to tell the doctor they are still feeling withdrawal and need a higher dose. They ask for an increase. Or they can cut back on their daily intake (remember, it has fewer withdrawal symptoms) and have extra to sell. I have heard from clients who easily decreased down four wafers to two in a couple months without withdrawal symptoms. Cutting a methadone dose in half can take months, or even longer, depending on the level.

The Suboxone treatment was originally only supposed to last 90 days. Some doctors are enforcing this, some are not. As mentioned before, if the client is not doing the recovery work necessary, or is not able to change his/her life circumstances fast enough, relapse is more likely than not. If the person is still living in a crack house, or is still in a relationship with someone using drugs, or has to walk through a neighborhood (or fishing dock) crowded with drug trafficking, or has family members or friends still coming to the door offering drugs in exchange for a place to "hang out" and get high, there is little chance for long term sobriety.

Though some doctors are very aware of these problems, many others who are licensed for Suboxone treatment are not experienced working with addiction. Suboxone, like methadone, is more dangerous when used in conjunction with alcohol or with benzodiazepines. Any of these drugs can suppress a person's respiratory system, and the combination of them risks a fatal overdose. Doctors who are not experienced in addiction treatment may be too easily talked into making exceptions, and may not be vigilant about tracking the drug screens and counseling that are supposed to accompany the treatment. They may not be aware that the client is drinking, or is "supplementing" the prescribed benzo with additional pills from the street.

Doesn't this happen at methadone clinics also? Absolutely. That is the point. Clinics have far more safeguards in place, and usually see clients daily, or at least weekly, and, even so, they still have difficulties controlling abuses. Suboxone clients are often not seen between visits, which may be a month apart. It is no wonder that a physician working alone has problems preventing those abuses. In a study at Yale,

> *"...the findings indicate that the methadone treatment subjects remained in treatment significantly longer and achieved significantly longer periods of sustained abstinence and a greater proportion of drug free urine tests, compared with subjects who received buprenorphine."*
>
> *Schottenfeld, et al.*

The best thing about Buprenorphine--that it is easier to detox off of--is the thing that makes it easy to abuse.

Suboxone is a welcome new "tool" that we can add to our toolbox to help clients battle opiate addiction. It works well for motivated clients who have their lives on track, and have a good, long clean time. It is a healthy step away from the structure of the clinic, back to a "normal" lifestyle. It is especially helpful for working clients, who fear that they will lose their jobs if they are seen on a methadone clinic, or are applying for a new job and fear the employer will test for methadone as well as illicit drugs. But it is not a replacement for methadone treatment.

3. *"Methadone doesn't work--Nobody ever gets off the clinic."*

"Do they have to stay on that stuff forever?"
Some do.
Some don't.
In my experience, there are three kinds of clients who have difficulty getting off the clinic successfully.

1. *These clients may want to stay on the clinic, but feel they have to keep their dose low and start detoxing as soon as possible, because they are being shamed by others to get off of it —*

Family, friends, doctors, Social Services workers, and probation officers may try to get them to get off of methadone: *"Aren't you off that stuff yet?"* Or the clients are afraid they will lose their reputation or their job if anyone finds out they are on it. They may have an open court case and be afraid they will be put in jail and be sick from methadone withdrawal. They often feel ashamed of their choice of treatment. They never give themselves a chance to stabilize and are likely to relapse sooner rather than later. They may get off of methadone, but most start using heroin or pills before they are even off the clinic, and they are back, too soon, with their lives still in chaos. When they get back on, they still have to hide it from their family or service providers, and they are again setting themselves up for failure.

2. *The second are the clients who resent the clinic, and see it as another authority trying to control them.*

This client gets angry at the rules as soon as they get on the clinic, and they can't wait to get off of it. They have heard all the bad things about methadone, and are ready to believe them. They also detox too quickly, and start getting sick. At that point, they will begin using illicit drugs again, and jump off the clinic, or are "thrown off" for non-compliance, only to come crawling back for another try. More recently, they may jump on to Suboxone, until they are thrown off of that for noncompliance. (The doctors who follow the buprenorphine protocol take drug screens and will terminate treatment of someone who is abusing opiates or other drugs.) Or, to stay on the clinic, they will have to go higher on their dose than they were before, because they have increased their tolerance level.

Every time someone goes back to the street drugs, then comes back to the clinic, or get themselves into serious withdrawal, by going down on their dose too fast, they will probably need a larger dose than before to feel "normal." They repeat the same pattern time after time. These are the clients who believe "you can't get off methadone without getting sick."

3. *And then there is the third kind of client. These people decide that they need the structure of the clinic, and don't trust that they can stay*

away from relapse without methadone.

They quietly put their lives back in order after the devastation resulting from their history of addiction. They do not trust themselves to be without the support. They don't believe their knowledge of the consequences of illicit drugs will be enough to keep them clean. I always hope that these clients will eventually feel stronger about themselves, but realize that they know better than I do. And until they feel confident that they are ready to slowly detox, pushing them to get off the clinic will cost more to them in anxiety and probable relapse, and will cost more to the taxpayer than leaving them on the methadone, even if they never do get off of it.

I would refer anyone interested in validating the need for long term methadone treatment to the NIDA (National Institute of Drug Abuse) report titled "Methadone at Forty",

> *"We now know that opioid dependence is a chronic disease, so we no longer think of methadone as a short term bridge to recovery, but instead consider it an intervention that may be beneficial indefinitely."*

People ask me, "What is the 'success rate' of people getting off the clinic?"

"Success" is not just people getting off methadone, but also keeping them off illicit drugs and ceasing illegal activity. For some, success means being able to get back to education or vocational training (with or without the methadone). Admittedly, the percentages look discouraging because we hope that people can end the treatment and get on with their lives. For most, this may not happen; but, contrary to popular belief, some people are able to do just that.

Getting off methadone voluntarily was rarely talked about as a realistic goal when I started work in 1996, even though we were required to put it in the yearly treatment plan as an eventual goal.

One of my clients showed me it was possible. She had done it before, then relapsed after some years of being clean (ran into an old boyfriend, as I recall). She jumped right back into treatment before she threw herself into financial ruin again. She got the relapse under control, and got off the clinic again fairly quickly. (By quickly, I mean in "Methadone time." She was probably there for at least 18 months.) She did it the right way: going more slowly as the dose decreased, (which is just when most clients decide they can go faster), and it worked for her. The last I saw her was a couple years later at an open house at her daughter's high school, and she looked great and said she was still working and staying clean. I knew, then, that getting off methadone without getting sick is possible. I shared her success story with other clients.

Quite a few clients have successfully come off the clinic in the past few years, some with a little help from Suboxone, others by going down on their dose slowly enough so they didn't get sick (The Narcan in Suboxone makes the jump from methadone to Suboxone difficult). Others are stable and continuing to go down slowly. The more they see others doing it the right way and not suffering withdrawal, the more they are encouraged to try. This is a good example of how group treatment can sometimes work better than individual sessions. This should not be a contest, however. It must be done from a position of choice and inner strength, not because they, or someone else, believe they "should" get off the clinic.

Shame is not a productive or effective way to motivate change.

These clients that are able to detox should be encouraged to continue their counseling and their group support after getting off the methadone. Relapses are the norm, and the more support available, the better their chance of success. And if relapse occurs, and they know that methadone treatment works for them, they can jump back on it soon enough to get their habit under control before too much damage has been done. The important thing here is to try not to get bogged down by shame that they have relapsed, which keeps them using in secret and is likely to prolong it.

Most counselors have seen clients who are able to get off the clinic.

People don't generally know about these clients, because they are not the ones hanging around badmouthing the clinic. They don't advertize their history, because they don't want to be judged on heroin's or on methadone's unsavory reputation.

4. *"The clinic just wants to keep clients there for the money."*

This belief is held by many clients, as well as many health professionals. It also arises from the reality, discussed above, that many people do stay in treatment for many years. Each time a client tries to pull off methadone too fast and fails, they are likely to need a higher dose than before to feel "normal." They experience frustration at going up on their dose when their intention was to get off the clinic. Sometimes the dosing staff gets blamed, not the fact that they tried to detox faster than the staff recommended.

This is not a perfect system. I'm sure there are programs and counselors that look too much at the bottom line. Like any business, the administration has to make sure the bills and payroll are covered. Keeping the numbers of clients up helps that bottom line.

Substance abuse counselors at clinics are not highly paid, and it is a difficult and often thankless job. Paperwork is overwhelming and relentlessly increasing every year. It's easier to have clients that we already enjoy working with, than starting with new.

Counselors can be guilty of assuming that clients will always need their help, and the structure of the clinic. Counselors are all too human, and everyone likes to feel needed.

Clients, who may feel safe with the support, can be forgiven if they resist giving it up. Change is scary.

We, both staff and clients, can get comfortable, and sometimes progress takes more energy than we can muster. Change is more difficult than staying in a rut.

But are we, as "the Clinic," conspiring to hold clients hostage? There are plenty of clients to go around. I see no shortage of new addicts, and plenty of returning ones.

The real problem is one of inertia on the part of clients and staff, not a devious intention to keep people on the clinic. If we discourage a person from detoxing themselves off the clinic, it is most likely because we believe that they are not ready.

I try to convey to clients that they never have to agree to a dose increase. The dosing nurse will offer an increase, based on what they know, what that client is telling them, and what they have learned working with others, but the decision is up to the client.

The only reasons we will usually recommend that the client up their dosage are first, the client is still using illicit opiates, or second, the client is complaining of feeling withdrawal symptoms.

Clients sometimes associate any feelings of discomfort to be a sign of withdrawal. If a client believes that going up on their dose will help them feel less depressed, the power of that belief might make it true. If the feelings of nausea or hot flashes or skin crawling are from a new medication, or from a cold or flu virus, they may think it is their dose, and decide to go up. There is also about a three-day lag between someone going up on the dose and their feeling the whole impact of that increase. They want instant relief from the increase, but three days after, they may come in "nodding" because it was more than they needed. Then I will encourage them to get another evaluation and go back down a little.

So, between clients' frustration regarding their inability to get off the methadone, and the factors of inertia that drive most aspects of our lives, it may look to some that the clinic wants to keep them there.

Where there is a problem of letting people stay on methadone longer than necessary, it can be helped by education, incentives, and lots of support on the part of staff and clients alike.

But please believe that there are plenty of addicts to go around. I do not lose sleep over not being able to keep clients on methadone. More to the point, there is a great sense of support, excitement, and encouragement among the whole staff when they see someone do well and get off the clinic successfully.

5. *"Heroin is worse than pills."*

There are opiate pills...

"I just did pills; I didn't do any hard drugs like heroin."

If someone starts with illicit opiate pills, or starts overusing their prescribed pain killers, it's just a matter of time. Some people begin with prescribed drugs after surgery. Some get pills from friends. Sometimes family members pass them out: "Here, take this, it will help your headache," or kids discover their grandmother's prescription box.

People ask, "How can some people take pain killers from their doctor and then get off of them while others become addicted?" This has a lot to do with whether the person learned healthy coping skills to manage discomfort as they were growing up. If someone saw their adult caregivers numbing their discomfort with alcohol or prescription medications, or was taught that they should not have to feel discomfort, or learned that discomfort is something terrible, and that they must rely on something outside themselves to help them feel better, then they will have a difficult time getting through the ups and downs of life without turning to the drug of choice for comfort. We'll look at this more when discussing pain management, in chapter five.

Plenty of clients at the clinic have never used heroin. They have gotten addicted to pills. The lawsuit won against the makers of Oxycontin shows how big a problem this has become. Addiction to opiate pills is physically the same as to heroin.

Does this make one client "better" than the other? Many clients find it helps their shame of being on methadone to think of themselves as "above" the heroin addicts. If the person had not gotten into treatment as soon as they did, they most likely would've been using heroin before long. Not many can afford the pill habit for long. It's just a matter of time.

Then there are benzodiazepines...

Benzodiazepines are another story. These are some of the most popular drugs around. If the generic name doesn't sound familiar, they are better known as Klonopin, Valium, Ativan, Serax, Xanex, and Librium. These are the same "Mother's Little Helper" pills passed out by doctors to my mother's generation to deal with "empty nest" problems.

They are wonderfully effective for short term use for anxiety, including panic attacks. And they are extremely addictive, both physically and psychologically.

These, in my opinion, are among the most abused drugs,

prescribed or illicit. They are most often responsible for clients who are seen dozing and drooling, or walking into walls, or stopping mid-sentence and having mental "time-outs" before becoming aware of their surroundings again- **The "Zombie" effect.**

These pills are a downfall for many people seeking recovery.

Benzos are one of the most disputed parts of methadone treatment, or other substance abuse treatment. Many clinics simply say their clients cannot be on any benzodiazepine while they are on methadone. The combination of benzodiazepines and methadone has resulted in many deaths.. If a dosage of these two drugs is too high, an individual can actually forget to breathe.

In my years at the clinic we have gone through waves of varying strategies as a new medical director may decide there will be no benzos allowed for methadone clients. The affected clients are thrown into panic over being forced off the pills, or they will try to get off the methadone, rather than give up their benzos. They will point out that the clinic was the one who originally prescribed them. They will claim they have been on them 30 years and so are sure that they cannot live without them. The clinic will then start eliminating the benzos, detoxing clients who are on them, and not allowing scripts by other psychiatrists. And then there will be one exception, then another. Within a year or so, the few exceptions will start to snowball, there will be multiple clients walking around (or stumbling) in a daze, and we will start all over again.

One problem is that a lot of addicts have very real anxiety

disorders, which is often a primary reason why they got into drugs in the first place. Benzos are the only drug that will quickly (and legally) take the edge off a panic attack.

There are a few clients who are able to take their script as prescribed, and it seems unfair to deny them this comfort. Unfortunately, for most, the script is an invitation to that longed-for high, where they escape from their intolerable feelings for a while. They take one extra pill, then four instead of two, and finally they take them by the handful, and this leads to the Zombie effect.

The National Institute on Drug Abuse reported that emergency medical visits for benzodiazepines outnumbered those of any other type of psychotropic agents in 2005.

We will talk more about this in the discussion of anxiety treatment.

Personally, I would rather work with someone high on heroin than someone heavily into benzos.

And then there are the non-narcotic pills...

Recently I have seen some methadone clients who look good "on paper." That is, they pass their urine screens, and if they have prescribed benzos, the level of benzo in their urine is within acceptable range. So why are they still looking like zombies?

Of course, the first thing to rule out is if the urines they are giving are "bogus", in other words, they are sneaking in "clean" urines instead of giving their own. This has become more possible because of budget cutbacks, where the client is left unsupervised while they give their urine. But, even supervised, many clients can get past the urine tests (if you don't know how, don't ask- it's not a pretty picture).

But if the client is not giving "bogus" urine samples, there are ways people learn to get around the tests. There are plenty of legal prescriptions which cause drowsiness without showing up on a drug screen. Besides the "sleeping pills" such as Ambien, there are the decongestants and cough formulas. Plenty of the psych drugs that are regularly (and appropriately) prescribed to these clients can be taken in excess to get the desired "nod". There are plenty of clients who are prescribed Seraquel or clonidine and can spare a few (for money).

And then there is the trick of taking "street" methadone on top of your prescribed dose, because the urine screen does not show the level of the dose.

Never underestimate the ingenuity of someone seeking to get high.

6. *"Heroin is worse than cocaine."*

Like benzos, cocaine is one of the downfalls for clients on methadone maintenance. Clients often get off to a great start on the clinic, feeling motivated and staying clean, sometimes for months, and then the first "dirty" drug screen comes in for cocaine. That client is in trouble.

Despite cocaine's more acceptable, "sexy" reputation in many circles, for the addict, it pulls them down like quicksand. Many methadone clients say, "I never liked cocaine before, I hate the way it makes me feel. But I can't stop using it." This is the origin of the belief discussed later: "Methadone makes you crave cocaine." For someone who has been "self medicating" with opiates, who can no longer do that (because of the methadone), they still feel a terrible need to get high. Cocaine is often the drug they use.

Cocaine _is_ addictive.

When individuals relapse on cocaine/crack, and are about to get a "disciplinary detox" from the clinic for noncompliance, we cannot get them into an inpatient detox because the party line of the insurance companies is: "cocaine is not physically addictive." This means that there are no visible physical signs of withdrawal such as the sweating, vomiting and "shakes" of those coming off heroin or alcohol.

There may be no obvious physiological withdrawal symptoms, but studies have shown that what cocaine does best is basically train your brain to crave it. It changes a person's brain chemistry. The belief that cocaine is not physically addictive is based only on a convenient definition which lets insurance get out of paying for an inpatient detox. This is one of our treatment system's "penny wise and pound foolish" policies.

Clients who have done both cocaine and heroin say that when you get high on heroin, you feel comfortable---you can forget about your troubles, and "go away" for a while (At least until you begin to feel withdrawal). But between "hits" you can function. Many clients even keep their jobs, with some planning ahead, so they have enough to get through the day. What they say about cocaine is that, at most, they may get a few minutes of the high before the only thing they can think about is getting more cocaine.

Some say that there is no pleasure left in the drug after a while, only the "chase" and the instant paranoia.

Sometimes hallucinations accompany the paranoia. Some clients report the firm conviction that bugs were crawling under their skin while they were high on crack, and they've tried to burn the bugs with cigarettes, burning their own arms in the attempt. A client once came in to a session looking exhausted and dirty, claiming his apartment house had burned down the night before. He confessed that he had started it by falling asleep with a cigarette. About three years later he admitted he had actually been high on crack, and was using his lighter to burn the "snakes" crawling on the curtains.

This is a drug that may be fun for the first few times, but for most of my clients it is no longer fun. It is a compulsion that brings misery and shame. And yet they feel powerless to stop. Sounds like my idea of a nightmare.

Cocaine promotes prostitution.

People prostitute for heroin, but I have heard about it more commonly for cocaine. A young client who boasted that she had never "worked the street" didn't last long after she got into shooting cocaine.

Some young couples on the clinic smoke crack. The same boyfriend who is incredibly jealous of another man looking in the general direction of his girlfriend, will send her out to prostitute, and expect her to bring back the money so they can go get high. They may mutually pretend not to know what she is doing, but in reality few of the boyfriends are stupid enough to be that naïve, and they do not hesitate to use all the appropriate verbal slurs against the woman when they fight.

Cocaine is worse for health than heroin.

When someone is on the methadone clinic and starts using, or relapses on cocaine, they start neglecting their health, missing appointments, not eating well. Often they stop taking necessary medications. They may supplement with heroin to "come down" and with benzos to ease the anxiety and paranoia aroused by the cocaine.

They again expose themselves to risky behavior through sexual contact and sharing paraphernalia (Snorting through straws can carry many viruses just as needles can). Cocaine enables the HIV virus and Hepatitis to multiply by lowering the immune system.

With cocaine use, mental health deteriorates, and panic and chronic anxiety come back full force. "What goes up must come down": the high of cocaine is followed by the crash of depression, especially when the person is already ashamed of their relapse, and they again find themselves sick, exhausted, and broke.

Cocaine messes with the methadone level.

A client metabolizes methadone more quickly if they are using cocaine. They will then need to go up on their dose to avoid opiate withdrawal symptoms.

Cocaine is harder on finances than heroin.

Heroin is one of the more reasonably priced illicit drugs,

at least when compared to pills and to cocaine (and even to pot). People can go through those lovely settlement or retroactive checks---thousands and thousands of dollars---in days with cocaine. And they do.

Cocaine is a destructive factor in methadone treatment.

If someone relapses on heroin, we can help them to stop by encouraging them to go up on their dose. If they relapse or start on cocaine, we only have the threat of throwing them off the clinic in an attempt to get them to stop.

We have been hearing that help is on its way, in the form of a drug that can block the pleasure from cocaine, as methadone does for heroin and other opiates. I've heard that the trial for one of these recently failed to test better than the placebo. NIDA website describes a trial for a vaccine that is still being tested.

Unfortunately, I have an uneasy feeling that if that option is put in place, the people who are still chasing that high will be going to whatever drug will top the cocaine, most likely methamphetamine.

7. *"Heroin is worse than alcohol."*

Alcohol is a part, not only of our culture, but of almost every culture. I sincerely believe that the first civilizations were built on the fact that early man saw it was worth giving up their relatively carefree nomadic hunter-gatherer lifestyle in order to cultivate grain to brew mead or grow grapes and make wine.

Recently there have been some health benefits proven for very moderate drinking habits, *but:*

Alcohol can be just as devastating to people's lives as heroin, contributing to domestic violence, child abuse, and chronic health problems.

The only advantage of alcohol abuse over heroin seems to be that the person who drinks is not automatically a criminal. Other than that, alcohol can be equally destructive. Both addictions progress over time, and both have serious health consequences. Both have devastating effects on the family of the addicted individual.

On the other hand, most of the domestic violence, the physical abuse, child molestation and sexual abuse I hear about is not a result of heroin addiction, but of alcohol abuse.

The majority of methadone clients in my women's domestic violence group tell me that unlike heroin, which tends to "mellow out" people (unless they are withdrawing); it is when their boyfriends drink that they are the most dangerous.

Many of my clients who, as children, were sexually abused, or severely beaten, or watched their mothers get beaten, state that alcohol was involved.

Don't get me wrong. I enjoy a glass of wine or an occasional cocktail. I am not advocating total abstinence and I am not interested in reinstating prohibition. I'm certainly not advocating legalizing heroin either. I'm just pointing out that thinking of one addiction as more morally deficient than another addiction is nonsense. This is not about morals.

This is about different unhealthy ways that people have learned to hide from their feelings and their problems.

8. *"People on methadone aren't 'clean.'"*

This is a phrase that my clients often are shamed with if they try to participate in the self help meetings in our area.

> ### Hostility often overtakes compassion in the recovery community.

In domestic violence training, we were taught the concept of "horizontal hostility." This is the idea that people who feel powerless will attempt to feel more empowered by seeing others (equally disempowered people) as even "less than" they are.

I often witness this concept in action within the methadone community as well. It happens at the clinic. People imply they are better than the "street junkie" by saying: "I never did heroin, I only did pills." Others brag: "I only sniffed it" or "I never stole for my drugs", or "I never stole from my family", and, finally, "I never worked the street." Many people will try to feel better about their own addiction by putting down others.

It's a human trait, if not a very honorable one.

Women who are afraid of losing their own children to DSS will call and report someone else's mistakes.
"Holier than thou" is a term my grandmother might have used to describe it. Whatever we call it, we all need to look hard in the mirror before judging someone else.

We all draw our line somewhere. If we step over that one, we tend to draw another one.

The recovery community, at least in our neck of the woods, often makes an unfortunate attempt to soothe the sting of their own problems by drawing the line at methadone. In many recovery programs, particularly AA and NA, the methadone client is shamed as "not clean." This is not a criticism of these very effective programs themselves, only of certain misuses of the original concepts by some individuals.

It's sad to see so many of the people struggling with addictions casting blame instead of lending support.

9. *"I hear people are dying from methadone overdose."*

Deaths of methadone clients have certainly risen in the past few years. Admittedly, this has been a problem, but again, it is more complicated than it first appears.

When someone who is on methadone dies of an overdose, many tend to assume it is the methadone that killed them. Many clients that have died on the clinic were also taking many other drugs, either prescribed or not. Again I would say benzodiazepines are often a contributing factor, especially when the client takes more than prescribed. This happens more times than most doctors realize.

Another important factor in the overall incidence of methadone deaths is the loosening of restrictions on prescribing methadone for pain.

Some doctors (often in pain clinics) who prescribe it may not be familiar with addiction or with methadone. The patient is given a bottle of the pills---they are not required to get their daily dose at a clinic. They get home and take the pills as prescribed. After a few hours they conclude that the dose is not helping, and they take some more. If they are not educated to understand that methadone is a drug that builds in their bloodstream over a period of several days, they may continue taking extra. When the full dose hits them, they are in serious trouble.

An article on Medscape Medical News reports finding *"poor correlation between dosages...and corresponding serum levels"* (methadone levels in the client's blood).

> *"We found people with very, very high dosages and low blood levels; and people with very high blood levels and low dosages, and the range was rather dramatic, actually...."*

> *"Their findings suggest that deaths that have been attributed to methadone because of high levels in their blood of the drug may not be after all the direct result of methadone overdose but rather the use of methadone in association with other drugs or underlying conditions."*

> *"The finger pointing at methadone per se appears to be a little misplaced."*
> > Medscape 2008: *Methadone Dosages Correlate Poorly with Serum Levels Susan Jeffrey*

Methadone clinics (with all their problems and shortcomings) are better structured to manage methadone than pain clinics or private doctors. We would all love to have easier solutions to opiate addiction and to pain, but opiate use for chronic pain is never going to be easy or simple.

10. "People on methadone don't need pain medication, since methadone is a pain medicine."

There is a lot of confusion about this one.

On the one hand, methadone was developed as a pain medication. Methadone is now given out (without the structured support of the clinic) at pain treatment centers.

Our clients are often told by doctors and dentists doing painful procedures that since they already take a pain medication, they shouldn't need more. My opinion is that if a client is used to their dose, then it provides little pain relief for acute pain.

Methadone is an opiate blocker, so a person on methadone maintenance has to use a lot more heroin or other opiates, if they want to "feel" the effect. Doesn't it make sense, then, that to medicate legitimate physical pain with opiates, the level would have to be increased? The individual already has a high tolerance for opiates; a prescribed opiate will be blocked at low doses by the methadone.

On the other hand, non-narcotic pain relief may be more effective and much safer for opiate addicted clients.

Even methadone clients have very different opinions of whether methadone maintenance helps chronic (long term) or acute (short term) pain management.

I have had clients almost off of methadone who decide it helps with chronic arthritis and other chronic pain issues, and they decide to go back up on their dose. Others say the methadone has no effect, and want to be treated with opiates. Others say that the non- narcotic pain relievers, like Motrin 800mg, help more for acute pain when they are on methadone.

I asked a doctor in charge of approving methadone treatment for Blue Cross clients whether he thought it worked for chronic pain management, and he said, "The jury is still out."

One of the confusing factors is the difficulty in distinguishing the power of the medication from the power of placebo effect. That can, of course, work both ways. If you believe something will help, then it is much more likely to help. If you believe it won't, it probably won't. This is true especially for something as subjective as pain.

The "drug seeking" client.

Most addicts are very sensitive to pain, and their threshold does not stop at their current dosage. If they have a tooth extracted, or get a hysterectomy, or have cancer, the dose is not likely to hold them for their pain. Do Percocet's help for their pain? I don't know, because I think it would have to be at a high enough dose to get "past" the blocking effect of the methadone. This could easily reach a dangerous level, because for anyone, opiate therapy can only do so much before the dose has to go up farther. This will be discussed in chapter five under "Rethinking pain management."

So does methadone maintenance work for acute pain? As

the doctor said, "The jury is still out."

But labeling a fellow human being, who has legitimate medical pain, as "drug seeking" is shaming and degrading, and is not good medicine. If they do not have physical pain, they most likely have emotional pain. And they feel completely helpless to control it without the medication they are seeking. They need to have those emotional needs acknowledged without the disgust that is often aimed at these clients. They need to be reassured that though the medication is not appropriate, there are ways they can control those overwhelming feelings.

Along with the rest of our society, they need to be educated that there are other ways to help physical pain besides pills, and that some pain is beyond our control, and has to be accepted as a part of life. But this can be done in a compassionate, not a punishing, critical, or disgusted way.

It is the addiction that has taken over a person's life like a parasite. It is the addiction that is the parasite, not the addicted.

CHAPTER TWO

Misinformation Addicts
tell each Other

A lot of the damage to methadone's "reputation" is perpetrated by the clients themselves, particularly by the ones who are eager to blame something or someone else---anything but themselves for their problems. Many clients arrive with a very well developed mistrust of authority figures, and are ready to believe what they hear in the parking lot rather than what the staff tells them. Other clients come into the clinic easily frightened by the "war stories" of why methadone doesn't work.

1. "Methadone is 'liquid handcuffs.'"

The clinic wants me to stay on methadone just for the money.

First: Don't worry; there are plenty of clients to go around-

Second: I guess your drug dealer was being charitable? Yes, I do need my paycheck, but I could also make three times the money doing private work. Addiction counselor is not a high paying job.

It is not the clinic controlling you. It is your addiction controlling you. If you really want to take back control of your life, stop blaming the people who can help you. Yes, the clinic has rules and, yes, your counselor has more power over you than you like- but the way to get your power back is to admit that you need those rules for awhile. You need that structure so that you can beat the real enemy, your addiction. You say that drugs made you feel free? That's the biggest lie your drug of choice tells you. It is a lie you are telling yourself. Maybe you have forgotten how you felt when you couldn't get them. The high doesn't come without the withdrawal.

"Liquid handcuffs" is another way to express the belief that the clinic uses methadone to control clients. The more control you get over your addiction, the less control the clinic will need to have over you.

"The addiction is the handcuffs."

Methadone is a key to those handcuffs, but the best clinic can only encourage your recovery. You are the one who has to do the work at freeing yourself. The more you try to "get over" on your counselor, or "beat" the drug screens, the tighter you are tying yourself to the clinic.

I hear of clients making fun of me for not catching them at lies, but I don't see that as an important part of my job. I am there to help people who want to help themselves. Getting over on the clinic or your counselor is hurting you, not them.

Being lied to on my job is, of course, to be expected. People lie for many reasons. Most often it is because they are ashamed of what they have done. Sometimes it is because they know they should be doing things differently, but they aren't ready to do that. Sometimes it seems like a compulsion. The people who are trying to outsmart the clinic will be the ones who don't make any progress and continue to blame everyone but themselves.

"They" keep me from getting off methadone by putting my dose higher and higher.

In the early days of methadone treatment, there was a limit to how high the dose could be. The dosing staff may be reacting against that outdated idea. We now know that the level is very individual. Remember, the therapeutic level can vary with changes in medications, levels of activity, and metabolism. HIV meds and Dilantin, among others, can cause the methadone dose to be used up faster.

Another drug that "eats up your methadone" is cocaine. Before the dose is increased, you should be clean for at least a week or two from cocaine, with no missed doses.

On the other hand, you should understand that you never have to agree to a dose increase. The dosing nurse will offer an increase based on what they know, on what you tell them, and what withdrawal symptoms they observe, but the decision is up to you.

> *An important note: The clients who refuse to go up on their dose when they really are still in withdrawal because they "want to get off fast" or have an idea that their dose shouldn't go over a certain number of milligrams are setting themselves up for failure. These are the clients I see fail time after time, getting off methadone. And they often relapse before they even complete their detox.*

The clients I see succeed are the ones that get on a comfortable dose, whatever that is (don't listen to your friends —listen to your own body). After being stable on that dose, and getting your life on track, then you can slowly go down on the dose. And, yes, it might take a couple years that way, but the point is, you will get off the clinic, and won't have to feel terrible doing it.

The choice is to rush off and almost certainly fail, or go slow and succeed. And if you are doing it the right way you will have your take-homes, so you will only have to go to the clinic every week or so anyway.

The reasons the staff will usually recommend that you go up on your dose are: 1-you are continuing to use illicit opiates, or 2- you are complaining of feeling withdrawal symptoms.

It's easy to associate any feelings of discomfort to be a sign of withdrawal. If you believe that going up on your dose will help you feel less depressed, the power of the belief might make it true. If the feelings of nausea or hot flashes or skin crawling are from a new medication or from a virus, you may think it is your dose and decide to go up.

Remember, with each relapse your tolerance for opiates increases, and so you will need a higher dose to feel "normal."

Again, I see clients fail who set a certain number of milligrams that they won't go over. Just because a certain dose was enough several years ago, does not mean it will be comfortable now. You may have increased your tolerance since then.

Clients will also shame other clients or see them as "just wanting to get high" if their dose is high. And yes, if the client is acting impaired, that could be true. But we now know that blood levels of methadone do not necessarily correspond to dosage. (*Susan Jeffrey*)

If the person does not seem impaired, they could be on a very high dose, and it may be appropriate. This can be checked by a blood test.

2. *"It eats your bones."*

I know you hear this from many other clients. It is not true. Most likely the belief comes from the fact that one of the very strong physical signs of withdrawal from opiates is aching bones.

The belief may be reinforced because when someone gets on methadone at 30 years of age and gets off at 45, they may find that those years, and possibly poor diet and little exercise, have taken a toll. Like the rest of us, their bones ache in the morning. The methadone, being a pain medication, has masked the aging and arthritis until the person detoxes.

> *"Methadone does not 'get into the bones' or in any way cause harm to the skeletal system."*
> New York: Drug Policy Alliance 2006

> *"If you are on methadone maintenance and you feel*

like your bones are 'rotting', it's probably because you're on too low a dose. Bone ache... is a symptom of methadone withdrawal"

CAMH

Every source I refer to states the same thing: There is no evidence that the methadone "gets in your bones", weakens them, "rots" or "eats" them. If your bones ache while on methadone maintenance you may be keeping your dose too low. If they ache when you are decreasing your dose, then it is a normal symptom of opiate withdrawal.

3. *"It rots your teeth."*

Again, I know how strongly many people believe this. And, again, it is not true. The problem is reinforced by the fact that while the person is "running"---using drugs daily and often other substances---they usually are not being careful to brush and floss daily, get regular cleanings, and eat healthy foods (There are a few exceptions, and these clients are much less likely to end up with dentures after getting into treatment). Many clients have phobias of dentists. They avoid them for years. The opiates they are using daily mask the pain as their teeth deteriorate. They get to the methadone clinic, and get on a maintenance dose, and are suddenly aware of the pain in their mouths.

Compounding this problem can be the fact that, as people move away from chasing drugs, they may turn to the more acceptable cravings of sweet coffee and soda and good old donuts.

One legitimate aspect of this myth which may be due to methadone is that, like many drugs, methadone can cause "dry mouth" *(CAMH)*. This can increase the chance of gum disease. Drinking plenty of water is, of course, a better solution than sucking on hard candy, although sugar free candy may relieve it without the damage.

Another huge factor many clients do not take into account is the role of cigarettes in gum disease and tooth decay. Many methadone clients are also heavy cigarette smokers. Cigarettes put the smoker at much higher risk for gum disease. Many clients object: "I gave up heroin; don't tell me I have to give up cigarettes."

It is far too easy to blame the methadone.

4. *"You'll get fat."*

Yes, you will see many clients gain a lot of weight when they get on methadone. No, it is not inevitable. Methadone does slow your metabolism some, but weight gain, with methadone clients just as with the rest of us, depends on taking in more calories than we use up.

Consider that before someone gets on methadone they are generally spending all their energy, time, and money supporting the opiate habit. They are not eating regularly, they are chasing the drug.

Then they get on the clinic. They no longer have to chase the drugs. Many have lost their jobs. Many have terrible histories of trauma from childhood and even more trauma after getting into drugs. They may have been suffering PTSD, depression, and anxiety since childhood. Those who haven't are just starting to deal with all the shame and the losses that are consequences of their drug use.

Many are unable to work or unable to find a job due to legal involvement. Others lack vocational training or social skills. Many have impulse control and anger problems which may have preceded their addiction. The way our current system works, it is easier for these clients---new in recovery---to at least temporarily get on welfare, sometimes on social security disability.

It is the exception when someone continues to work, and unfortunately many of these workers have more difficulty maintaining recovery, because of the demands of counseling and dosing schedules Some find that their work places are triggers to relapse (i.e. waitresses who find cocaine used regularly in staff bathrooms; fishing docks where the dealer is waiting as you get off the boat). These working clients also have more difficulty getting the insurance needed to help pay for the treatment. (Massachusetts has taken a step to alleviate this with the state wide health insurance)

And so, typically, many clients have no job to help them structure their daily schedule. Inertia often takes over. They can sleep in, or (as many clients do) they can go get their dose, then return home and watch their shows.

Many clients have no experience with healthy diet habits. The standard is often donuts and sweet coffee. It is easier and cheaper to eat poorly than to buy fresh fruits and vegetables. There are few incentives to exercise.

Many go on antidepressants, which also slow metabolism and make it even harder not to gain weight.

You combine lack of activity, a slowed metabolism, and a

poor diet, and guess what? The clients rapidly gain weight. This is closely tied to the next belief:

5. *"Methadone makes you crave sweets."*

Another misconception.
Or maybe I should say exaggeration.

Yes, methadone slows your metabolism and that donut seems like it will make you feel better.

I don't think methadone clients have a corner on craving sweets. What's my excuse? Sweets are a national weakness. Comfort foods, empty carbs are a habit. When we are anxious, depressed, or bored, our immediate thought is to go for the comfort foods.

When individuals are trying not to relapse, they are especially likely to do some emotional eating. And who can say what is right? I have encouraged some clients that it is healthier to fill that craving with cheesecake rather than cocaine, at least for awhile.

But this can be another place in which we take responsibility for our own behavior. We are still responsible for eating that whole box of cookies. Of course you want to, but you have a brain attached to that hand feeding you the cookies. What would you tell a three-year-old who wants to eat three desserts and no dinner? You'd tell them they can eat their (one) dessert after they eat their dinner. We need to tell ourselves that.

I have seen clients who take control of their weight issue. As for most of us, it is a difficult battle, but we can't blame it solely on the methadone.

6. *"Methadone makes you crave cocaine."*

And that brings us to another firmly held belief. Many clients start using cocaine when they get on methadone. I hear, "I never liked it before, I still don't like it but I can't stop using it." This is not a particular craving, but a substitute addiction. They cannot feel the "high" of dope because methadone blocks it, so they often turn to cocaine. That they can't stop using it is the nature of the cocaine, not the urge created by methadone. Other clients do not use cocaine, but find themselves getting high some other way, whether it is on benzodiazepines or drinking alcohol. Their need to get high is still there, even though the high of the opiate is blocked. The client is still looking for a way not to feel those uncomfortable feelings they continue to run from.

As a matter of fact, a recent study showed that lab rats were less attracted to cocaine if they were on methadone. You may have heard of the early experiments in which rats, given a choice to push a lever for food or for cocaine, would literally starve themselves, neglecting their own need for food in order to get more cocaine.

Now there is a study that shows if the rats are on methadone, they will use less cocaine.

> *"Continuously administered, high dose methadone undermined animal's motivation to acquire cocaine."*
> *NIDA Notes Volume 22, Number 2*

The "cocaine craving" is not a physical craving created

by methadone, but is a desire to continue to get high. Unfortunately, the general culture of the clinic presents ample opportunity.

7. *"It's harder to kick than dope."*

This one is, in many ways, true. Heroin withdrawal is over in 3-8 days. Methadone can stay in your system for a month.

The misunderstanding, though, is the idea that it is impossible to detox from methadone without terrible withdrawal. Some variations of this are:

"You have to get sick to get off of it."

This belief comes from people who try to detox from the methadone too quickly. Yes, it takes a long time. But if you try to rush, you are likely to end in failure. The lower your dose is, the larger a percentage each milligram is. So, at 100mg, you can take away 5mg and that is only taking away 5% of what your body is used to. At 10mg, if you take away 5mg, that means taking 50% of what your body is used to. Even taking 1mg from the 10 is taking 10%. So the lower your dose gets, the slower you need to go. For a population that generally has problems with impulsiveness, this may feel like torture to take so long. I usually recommend going down 1mg per month for the last 10 mg. And most clients I suggest that to say, "But that will take 10 more months!" And my reply is that if they try to move faster they are risking relapse, and are very likely to end up going back up on their dose (probably higher than before they started detoxing). So, take your choice: Do you want to be off the clinic after those ten months, or back where you started or on an even higher dose?

People forget how fast those 10 months will go.

Hopefully, when you are trying to detox you are already getting your take-homes. If you are not getting take-homes then most likely there are still issues you need to address before you should start detoxing. Are you still on benzodiazepines? Then you need to learn better ways to deal with anxiety. Are you still smoking pot? Maybe you should figure out why you still need that escape, before you try to give up the structure of the clinic. And that extra time might give you time to build your new life, to make social connections beyond the dealer and drug friends. Maybe it will provide time to get some vocational training or get back to your education.

It's far too easy an excuse to think you can't make a new life because the methadone clinic is holding you back. There are plenty of methadone clients who are devoting their time to living that new life, and they will have the advantage that when they are ready to slide off that last milligram of methadone (painlessly), they will not have dealers knocking on their door or someone in their life eager to help them relapse.

Each person handles withdrawal from methadone differently. There will be some symptoms as you detox, but those symptoms can be kept at a tolerable level,

"The only way to get off of methadone is to go to a detox."

I have not seen anyone successfully go into an inpatient

detox program to get off of methadone. Most detoxes give them benzodiazepines, and these can mask the withdrawal until the person is then released with no meds and still suffering withdrawal. The only situation in which this may work is if the person can go directly into a long term residential program. Unfortunately, there are few of these available. So the person is released with instructions to call for availability of a program, and the drug dealer meets them at the next corner.

It is possible to get off methadone without major discomfort. The ones who are still at the clinic telling you how impossible it is are the same ones who keep doing it wrong. The ones who do it the right way aren't still hanging around.

"Nobody ever gets off methadone without relapsing."

I wish I could tell you this was false. There are a few who make it off and years later are still doing okay, but, even these realize that it is possible to fall. I don't think they would tell me to put "never". Unfortunately there are many who do relapse: **Opiate addiction is not something you can fix and forget**. It is a chronic condition, ready to come back full force if given an opportunity. The best we can do, and the best you can do if afflicted by it, is to learn from mistakes, and never take your recovery for granted. Watch for the red flags, and keep the chance of relapse at a minimum. If you find a good counselor, make sure you check in with them. If you find meetings help you, keep those in your life.

And if you do relapse, get help as soon as you realize you

are having trouble. I have seen clients who have gotten off methadone, experienced some years of clean time---then they meet someone from the past, or go on opiate pills after surgery, and suddenly they realize they are back to old patterns. Their best option is to get back on the clinic, and (if they did it right the first time), they can soon stabilize and detox again.

The more insight they have into their own patterns, the more control they have.

8. *"I've heard 'they' can 'put you out' and filter your blood in one day to get off of methadone (or opiates)."*

This sounds great, but whoever is paying for it (poor old mom or dad?) better look at the odds before spending the $15,000 or more.

If the client hasn't done the "head" work they need to do, then the first stressful situation that the person faces, guess what is likely to happen? Maybe it is a reasonable option if you're a rock star, but not for the rest.

If getting through physical withdrawal was all that was needed to cure heroin or other opiate addiction, an eight day inpatient detox would do just fine.

As stated before, you probably know someone who was hospitalized for a couple weeks without their cigarettes. How many like these (even the ones who try to stay off of them) make it through the first stressful situation without reverting to "needing" that cigarette?

I've heard addiction described as a "worn path" in the way our brain works. The first thing that someone thinks of when they are stressed is to take that worn path, right to the drug of choice. It takes a lot of motivation and the hard work of learning healthier coping skills to be able to choose the new path.

And other alternative treatments

There is another experiment (it's been tried before) in Canada in which heroin is being legally injected for those who, despite treatment, still chronically use. My guess is that, if this treatment is accepted, we'll soon have a whole lot more people that think methadone doesn't work for them. And, there is still the problem with people's tolerance continuing to climb. At some point it becomes lethal. Also, in the article it was noted that there were a lot more "adverse incidents" with the injected prescribed heroin. This means more overdoses and seizures.
Cassel: Medscape, 2009

Narcan patches are also being tested as an alternate treatment. These show some promise, but are not yet widely available.

We would all love it if addiction could be fixed quickly, easily, cheaply. It can't.

9. *"I got on the clinic for opiates- it's none of their business if I do cocaine, alcohol or pot."*

My question to a client like this: "Why should the tax pay-ers or the insurance company feel obliged to pay for your methadone treatment so that you can still put yourself at risk with the other addictions?"

Heroin is actually in many ways easier on people's health than most of the other addictive drugs---even alcohol. If it weren't for the fact that tolerance develops with opiates, it would be great...but of course the tolerance does develop.

There are former clients that I will not encourage to get back on methadone. Their pattern is to develop a bad heroin habit on the street, and come onto methadone so they don't have to worry about being sick every morning. They then use this as an opportunity to go back to smoking crack or drinking.

Especially for those who have chronic infections such as HIV or Hepatitis, the cocaine or alcohol will do more harm than the heroin.

Another problem with the methadone clinic "looking the other way" at other drug or alcohol use is that the combi-nation can be lethal.

As mentioned before, both alcohol and benzodiazepines can increase the sedative effect of the methadone. Together they can depress a person's respiration and kill them. It would be bad medical practice to give out methadone and not worry about the other drug or alcohol use.

Pot, of course, is always brought up as the "harmless" drug. And yes, I usually do not push as hard for people to get off this as I do other drugs. The clinic used to give people "disciplinary contracts" for pot, and then decided to just require them to attend a marijuana group---to educate them on the long term health effects and encourage cessation. Now it is largely ignored unless their individual counselor chooses to work on it. The only consequence is that they can't get take-homes. These policies vary from clinic to clinic.

There is new research confirming that pot has some connection to more severe psychotic symptoms, and there are long term health effects. If nothing else, because it is less refined than tobacco, smoking pot is at least as bad or worse for people's lungs than cigarettes. And the newer "designer" pot is not only exorbitantly expensive, but much more likely to cause paranoia and to contain additives to "boost" the high.

I have seen people finally stop using pot after years of daily use. Sometimes it is a matter of motivation, to get their take-homes, or to go for a job they want. The people I have seen achieve this have reported not missing it nearly as much as they thought they would.

Beside reasons of health, I guess the reason I concern myself with trying to help people get off these other drugs is so they can find out that life can lived without the escape of a drug.

10. *"I just need the methadone, I don't need counseling," or -"Just give me my dose."*

A client who had been on the clinic on and off for many years told me that when he first entered treatment in the 70's, he took part in a clinical trial to see if just getting on the methadone would work without counseling. He said that after several weeks there were no clean urine screens among those without counseling.

A clinic that promotes treatment without strong social and psychological support is known as a "juice bar." Few clients who are seriously working on their recovery would recommend the "dose only" philosophy.

If you have legitimate problems with your counselor, talk to the program director about changing to someone you can talk to. There really is something to the importance of being "a good match" of client to counselor, and counselors (being human) can have their own issues. Then again, if you have switched counselors several times, and are still thinking it's the counselor's fault, maybe you'd better try to figure out what you are doing that is getting in the way of your progress.

Another problem is that there is a lot of "turnover" with substance abuse counselors. They often leave after a short period of time. Clients get tired of trying to open up to someone just to see them leave a few months later. I hope anyone feeling this will keep trying. Hopefully you can take lessons from each part of your journey.

11. *"I can't stand groups; everybody just tells 'war stories.'."*

This is a frequent complaint when we try and get people into group treatment. Insurance, of course, promotes group treatment. Obviously this would be convenient for the insurance company since group treatment is cheaper than individual sessions. But I've come to believe that, for a majority (not for every client), groups are an important part of recovery, sometimes more effective than individual sessions.

Many clients have had bad experiences with group treatment. I do not deny that groups can be badly handled. I made my own mistakes as I learned to run groups at the clinic.

But I have also seen the advantages of group treatment. There have been many cases where I, as therapist, did not see the interpersonal problems a client had until I saw them interact in a group. Clients can put on a convincing façade for a naive therapist, but they will not fool the other clients for long.

And clients are much more open to believe something a client tells them from first-hand experience.

Groups are much more efficient for teaching (and practicing) social and communication skills as well as anger management. The best thing about effective groups is, of course, for clients to realize that they are not the only ones who have gone through experiences similar to their own, and that others have felt what they are feeling.

12. *"My counselor never even used drugs– how can he/she help an addict?"*

This brings us to the next strongly held belief

Many clients are skeptical when they first meet me and question whether I will be able to understand their experience of street life and addiction, since I have not experienced it myself.
This was a good way to shake my confidence during my first couple years at the clinic. I understand their apprehension. The world I grew up in seems like another world. The world I go home to is a very different place than most of them still live in.

On the other hand, as a "foreigner" to "the street," I find I am able to be a more objective observer, without the preconceived notions of what "should" work. And I don't overuse the standard, stereotypical phrases that sometimes become so familiar as to lose their meaning. I believe clients are often relieved to receive a fresh view of how to approach their problems. I believe I may have a more realistic grasp of what my clients so often say they long for: a "normal" life. Yes, I know "normal" does not exist, but we can refer to a "normal range.": A life that does not revolve around substance/alcohol abuse and violence, police being called to break up family fights, and children thinking that going to jail is part of growing up.

I now know that it takes empathy to do addiction counseling. It requires a desire to help an individual, not experience in shooting up..

CHAPTER THREE

What Doesn't Work in Methadone Treatment

The old style of addiction treatment was to confront a client, often accuse him or her of being in denial, and demand abstinence or else suffer termination from treatment. This has been shown to be ineffective in many cases.

1. shaming

You'll never do a better job at shaming a heroin addict than what they do to themselves. The problem is (I can't remember who I am quoting) "shame doesn't promote change," and what we want is for the addict to be able to change. **Shame is more often a trigger to relapse than a reason to stay clean.** The thought goes: "Why try, I'm just a loser, I'm going to fail anyway. I may as well get high." Shame does not promote *long term* change.

I find that many people outside the drug community think that an addict must have been brought up with no discipline. *"The trouble is, they needed a good kick in the pants..."* Though it is sometimes true that the person did not appropriate rules enforced in their childhood (and possibly more often with the younger addicts), many that I have met were brought up in either very strict, or at least very punitive or critical homes. Many were regularly beaten. Some were abused throughout their childhood, whether physically, emotionally, verbally, or sexually. Many were considered from a very young age (sometimes from birth) as the "black sheep" of the family, and were treated as outcasts.

Even those who say their parents were very loving are struggling with all the shame they feel for hurting their loved ones.

The person thinks, "I don't deserve to get better, I've hurt too many people." Humiliation and shame are all too familiar, and the only way they know to make that shame go away (momentarily) is to continue to use drugs.

Rational? NO, but one of my most reliable rules for understanding people's behavior is to realize that: PEOPLE ARE NOT RATIONAL. We all want to believe we are rational, but WE ARE EMOTIONAL, with a *very* thin veneer of rationality on top.

One thing most addicts have is a very strong "Rebel" voice in their head. If you try to force treatment or try to shame them into giving up their drug of choice, they may have a strong part of themselves that wants very much to stay clean, but that "Rebel voice" will win just about every time. This is true of most of us. Truthfully, when someone looks down at you and says "You'd better do this my way, or else," isn't your first instinct to say "Oh yeah? I'll show *you*"?

One of the most harmful ways this shame is played out is when clients are afraid to share with their doctors that they are on methadone. Unfortunately, often this fear is warranted. I've heard too many very good people tell me that as soon as they tell the doctor they are on the clinic, the doctor's attitude changes. I always encourage them to find a doctor who is sympathetic (not enabling) of addiction. There are some very good knowledgeable doctors who do understand.

2. *When well intentioned people try to push clients to get off the clinic...*

This is one of the most destructive dynamics that under-mines progress in so many clients.

First, to get off of methadone successfully, the client needs to feel safe. They have to have a stable enough income/insurance to pay for treatment. *(You might think, "but they found the money for their dope". Yes, but we don't want them stealing or scamming or prostituting for their treatment.)*

Then they need to take care of old legal issues, get on psych meds if needed, and take care of medical problems, find new social outlets, and then (the hardest) find new ways to cope with people and their own emotions, so they do not relapse at the first trigger.

They need to figure out, "If I am not a drug addict, who am I?"

If you know someone on methadone, you do not know when they need to get off the clinic. Even if you have been on methadone; you may not know what is best for someone else. Talk to them, encourage them, but try not to insist that you know what they need more than they do.

If you are a methadone client, don't let people push you to go down on your dose too fast, or to even start trying to detox until you have a good long clean time and feel confident that you are ready.

If someone rushes down on their dose too quickly, they can get into serious physical withdrawal, and then their choice is usually to start "supplementing" their dose with pills or street drugs, or go higher on their dose than they were before they started their detox.

This is a case of, **"Is what you are doing getting you what you want?"** (the reality principle). If you want your friend or family member to get off of methadone, pushing them to start detoxing before they are really ready will end up increasing their time on the clinic (or back on the street).

If you are a methadone client, and people are pressuring you to get off the clinic before you feel ready, please know that this has to be a decision you and your counselor make. Methadone is a legal medicine. Listen to your own body. Although someone might find a reason not to hire you because of methadone, they cannot fire you as long as you are not coming to work impaired.

Your DSS/DCF worker may threaten that you will not get your kids back if you are on the clinic but this is not true. If your family judges and shames you for being on methadone, then you don't need to share the details of your recovery with them.

3. Time limits on treatment.

When the Massachusetts State legislature was debating funding for methadone treatment (I was quoting one of them with the phrase "methadone junkies"), they discussed setting a time limit on methadone treatment. We heard all kinds of rumors. Someone suggested a time limit on each admission to the methadone clinic. "Get them on, get them off..."Another suggested limiting how many times a person could be admitted in their lifetime.

The result would have been even more failed treatments. Clients get anxious enough trying to get off the stuff, without mandated time limits. The more pressure to get off the clinic, the more chance they will fail, or relapse trying. If, as some proposed, there was a lifetime "cap" on times in treatment, I fear there would not be more efficient use of their treatments—to the contrary, there would be more desperation and lost options. I have had some clients in treatment for years suddenly find that they are stable enough to slowly detox from the clinic. They will tell you that if they had tried before that time, they would've failed.

When a client's family, doctors, probation officers, or DSS/DCF workers push them to get off of methadone you get the same reactions. Remember, addiction is not about intellectual understanding. Most addicts are painfully aware of the devastation they are causing themselves and their families. Addiction is partly physical, but much stronger than that is the part that is purely emotional. It is the only way most addicts know how to stop the overwhelming negative feelings that they believe are intolerable: "If I couldn't get high, I'd kill myself to stop feeling what I feel."

We now know from numerous studies that the longer we can keep someone in treatment, the more likely we can reduce the harm they do to themselves (and their family and the community), and the more likely that they will finally be able to "get it right."

4. *Limits on dose.*

When methadone treatment began, there was often a limit to how high the dose could go. I have heard that 100 mg was deemed sufficient for everyone. Unfortunately many factors vary between individuals. Metabolism, level of activity, and medications can influence how fast someone metabolizes their dose. It is the therapeutic level, not the number of milligrams taken, which keeps someone from feeling withdrawal. Someone feeling those withdrawal symptoms will have much more difficulty functioning well, whether it is taking care of a family, or working at a job. They will also be much more likely to "self medicate."

We now know that the effectiveness of a dose level for each individual is not simple arithmetic. A study presented at the American Academy of Pain Management, states:

> *"We found people who had very, very high dosages with low blood levels, and people with very high blood levels and low dosages, and the range was rather dramatic, actually."*
> *Medscape: Methadone Dosages Correlate Poorly*
> *with Serum Levels*

Another research team wrote:

> *"Each patient presents a unique clinical challenge,*

and there is no way of prescribing a single best methadone dose to achieve a specific blood level as a 'gold standard' for all patients. Clinical signs and patients reported symptoms of abstinence syndrome, and continuing illicit opioid use, are effective indicators of dose inadequacy." There does not appear to be a maximum daily dose limit when determining what is adequately 'enough' methadone in MMT (Methadone Maintenance Therapy)"

When " 'Enough' is not Enough" Leavitt, et al

A warning to methadone providers: Be particularly cautious of very large doses with take-homes- We had an incident in which someone who had a very large dose, a lot of take-homes, and a good clean record, turned out to be selling a sizeable portion of his dose. The only way we found out was that a former client almost died and her boyfriend called and reported who had been selling her his methadone.

Many clients are comfortable on doses from 60-120mg daily, but many need much more to feel comfortable. And some can go lower after they are stable, and keep it at just enough to prevent themselves from giving in to temptation.

5. *Dosing without counseling.*

As discussed in the previous chapter, one of my clients had been in and out of methadone treatment since it began. He told me that he volunteered to be in a study on whether counseling made a difference to successful treatment. He was one that received dosing, but was not required to give urines or be in individual or group counseling. He reported that at the end of the study, every one of the clients in his group was still using.

I was reminded about this by a recent headline on AOL announcing that a "miracle pill" may end alcoholism. The response from the Betty Ford Center stated that the assumption shows that the reporter doesn't understand the complexity of the addiction. The AOL article then commented, "of course, because their jobs, as well as bartenders' jobs would be threatened." Somehow I don't think rehab directors (or definitely bartenders) will be put out of business anytime soon, no matter how many "miracle pills" they come up with. Methadone is a great example which underlines the fact that addiction is not that easily fixed.

The reason for this is connected to the next aspect of treatment that doesn't work:

6. *Treating the addiction without treating the psychiatric problem.*

I have met very few clients at the methadone clinic who do not qualify as "dual diagnosis" clients. This means that they have at least one substance abuse diagnosis, and also meet the criteria for another mental disorder. Some of the most common are:

ADHD
Bipolar Disorder
Borderline Personality Disorder
Depression
Generalized Anxiety
Obsessive Compulsive Disorder

> Panic Disorder
> PTSD (Post Traumatic Stress Disorder)
> Schizophrenia
> Social Phobia

And, yes, some people acquire these disorders after getting into drugs, but that doesn't make them less real for that person. These become the reasons a quick detox does not work.

And I believe that for a majority of people, the problems they have with the mental health issue came first, and it is often what makes them vulnerable to becoming seduced by the drugs in the first place.

This is not the place to go in-depth on these mental disorders, but a brief explanation of why they may make people susceptible to substance abuse is appropriate.

ADHD

There is plenty of controversy about this diagnosis. Many parents don't want their children medicated because they feel this will make them more likely to abuse drugs later in life. Studies are showing this belief is unfounded--that kids who are treated young are neither more nor less likely to abuse drugs. Unfortunately the diagnosis itself is a risk factor for substance abuse, whether treated or not.

I also have mixed feelings about putting kids on medication. I've written more about this in my book, Generation RX, Kids on Pills. I do know that, for some kids, treatment helps them in school, and prevents the child from being labeled "bad." I am also very aware that at this time many young people are getting their first highs off of ADHD medications.

I believe that sometimes anxiety symptoms, trauma related symptoms, and behavioral problems can be interpreted as ADHD.

I believe that many children who did get labeled as problems in school, and did not receive the help they needed to succeed in schoolwork have gone on to "self medicate," whether with pills, pot, or alcohol.

Bipolar Disorder

Originally the name was "manic-depressive". Again, this is a diagnosis that was considered unusual until a few years ago. Now it seems three quarters of the clients on the clinic have been told at some point that they are Bipolar.

And, even scarier, far too many kids are now diagnosed with it.

Many times there is some confusion about what the diagnosis means. I will hear, "Yeah, I'm Bipolar---one minute I'm really down and the next minute I'm going crazy." This is not the criteria for a Bipolar diagnosis. What that person is describing is mood swings. Bipolar (at least the original definition) is more correctly described as at least one major depressive episode with symptoms lasting over a two week period, and then at least one distinct episode of "mania," with "inflated self esteem or grandiosity," "increase in goal oriented activity," sometimes with decreased need of sleep, racing thoughts, and often excessive high risk behaviors. This manic episode must last at least a week to meet the original diagnostic criteria.

The Bipolar diagnosis has been expanded and now has some variations, which account for the recent "boom" in numbers. I heard recently that the Bipolar diagnosis has increased something like 4000% in the past twenty years.

The classic Bipolar symptoms are extremely destructive to the client and to their families. This diagnosis is often seen in families with a history of severe emotional abuse, often sexual abuse.

The risky behavior of the manic phase often involves substance abuse.

Borderline Personality Disorder

This diagnosis was considered "politically incorrect" for awhile, because it was mostly used to label women, and was one of those "I know it when I see it" diagnoses, in which specific criteria to pin it down were difficult to identify.

As with Bipolar, it is often associated with early abuse, especially incest. People diagnosed with this are often extremely volatile emotionally, may make frequent suicide attempts, or perform self harming behaviors like cutting. They may become your instant best friend, and then the next day they decide you are their worst enemy. They can be very high functioning and intelligent (or not). They can keep their lives in constant chaos, as well as the lives of those around them.

Emotional ups and downs (those mood swings), and extreme impulsivity are part of this diagnosis, and make an easy connection to substance abuse.

Depression

This is a problem that may come as a consequence of getting involved with drugs or alcohol. When individuals try to get their life back on track, they will have to face all the harm they have done to themselves and to anyone close to them. They may have lost their marriage, their kids, their home. They may have wrecked their health. Who wouldn't become depressed?

Often people were depressed before they started using drugs. The drugs became the way they could feel better. I hear many women say, "The only time I've ever liked myself is when I'm high."

I try to distinguish depression from **bereavement**. Many depressive episodes begin with grief. If someone still needs to grieve, no antidepressant is going to make things better. Someone with a severe loss who goes quickly into substance abuse to cover up those intensely uncomfortable feelings will still need to do the grief work before they can give up their drug of choice.

Generalized Anxiety

Some people are always anxious. They are probably (literally) born anxious. They are always thinking the worst is going to happen, that something terrible is just around the bend. Drugs and alcohol provide some welcome relief, until that substance becomes the problem. People who suffer from anxiety need to learn better ways to calm themselves so they don't relapse on the substance.

Obsessive Compulsive Disorder

This is incredibly common among the clients I meet at the methadone clinic. It is a relentless disorder in which nothing but perfection will do, and of course, there is no such thing as perfection. Again, drugs seem to provide relief, at least temporarily.

Panic Disorder

Panic attacks are characterized by the heart thumping, dizzy feeling, I-can't-breathe attacks that are triggered by some situation or thought, and can cripple people as they give over their life to fear, limiting themselves more and more as they try to avoid anything that might trigger another attack. Then it becomes an additional diagnosis of **Agoraphobia** (the fear of fear).

Even someone who would never think of seeking out a drug to get high will be given benzos by their family doctor if they report these symptoms. If they are not careful, they may become dependent on them.

PTSD (Post Traumatic Stress Disorder)

Many of the clients I see have been exposed to trauma from birth (some even before birth). Some of the hardest kinds of trauma to treat are the chronic (daily) fears that a child lives within an abusive and/or addicted home.

Others have a relatively "normal" childhood but then experience a tragedy of a violent death of a family member, or are themselves in a fearful accident, or are attacked or raped. War, of course, is another cause of PTSD. Not everyone who experiences these hardships gets PTSD. This depends on the particular incident, the age of its occurrence, and on the person's coping skills. Those who are not well equipped with coping skills and close support are likely to develop PTSD. This means that waking and sleeping, they have to constantly relive the feelings of that traumatic moment. People will do a lot, including drugs they know are harmful, to avoid those flashbacks.

Once involved in the drug world, they are likely to be exposed to many more traumatic events. It becomes harder for the person to ever feel "normal", or feel that returning to a "normal" life is even possible.

Schizophrenia

This is the classic diagnosis of the "street person." The criteria usually involves serious psychotic symptoms, often "hearing voices", which tell the person to harm themselves or others. It is much more controllable with the new antipsychotic meds, though it remains one of the most chronic and devastating mental health diagnoses.

Social Phobia

This is the diagnosis characterized by crippling shyness from early childhood. These children have problems with standing up in front of their class in school, and often fear blushing or humiliation if they are the center of attention. They may have problems with stuttering. They will be limited by this condition in school and, later, in their job. Many clients report getting high was their first experience of feeling comfortable in a social situation. I remember a man who depended on alcohol: who said, "I would stop at the liquor store on the way to a party to 'pick up my personality'."

Alcohol and drugs may offer welcome, if temporary, relief from fears and discomfort.

Anger Problems

One very common symptom we see at the clinic, which keeps a lot of clients from progressing, is explosive anger. This does not have an official diagnosis in the current DSM4, (The manual used to diagnose people), but is likely to be recognized in the upcoming edition. So the symptoms are placed under **"Intermittent Explosive Disorder"** or, usually appropriately, as part of the PTSD symptoms. These behaviors make it difficult for the client to get along with people, especially anyone in authority. The client usually does not realize that he or she may have something to do with the world feeling so hostile. And, as usual, when someone is angry, often the best solution they know is to get high.

This is, of course, a problem with many people today, not just methadone clients. But impulsive anger and chronic rage, often with violent behavior, undermines progress. People with anger problems tend to believe that the world (or the clinic) is out to get them, and so they are always ready to attack rather than wait to be attacked. Having lived in an abusive home, in jail, and/or "on the street" has confirmed their belief that "it's me against the world."

I have met few clients on the clinic who are not "dual diagnosis." Without sufficient treatment of these problems, long term recovery is precarious at best.

7. *Allowing other addictions to replace the opiates (including legally prescribed drugs)*

Whether it is cocaine, alcohol, benzos, or over-the-counter meds, long term recovery is unlikely if the person still depends on some kind of "altered state" to cope with the bumps in the road.

There are, of course, some habits that are healthy. Even these can become unhealthy if the person goes to extremes: Exercise is a classic example. Exercise is proving to be more helpful to improve depression than psychiatric medications. While I encourage my clients to find an exercise routine that works for them, many of the clients I work with can't do anything without overdoing it.
This is the unhealthy "all or nothing" mind set. Exercise can become a symptom of anorexia if the person uses it as a "punishment" for overeating.

I have been known to indulge in treating myself to shopping when I'm feeling down. As long as I stay within my means, and have other coping skills available to me, I don't see it as a problem. If I got to the point in which I had to start hiding my purchases and couldn't handle the credit card payments, I would consider that a problem.

As a therapist (and I try to apply this to myself as well as my clients) I want to look at the "overall picture."

I began as an English major in college. One of the main themes throughout English literature (actually it originated with Plato, I believe)is "the Golden Mean." It's about keeping a balance in life. When we go to extremes, we get into trouble. When our sense of worth depends on a certain body weight, or a certain person loving us, or a certain job or level of income, then we are out of balance. When we can't face the existential realities of life (and death), and have to medicate ourselves to deal with them (or distract ourselves with endless TV or constant technical or social distractions), then we're in trouble. If all our energy goes into one area of our life and we neglect the other parts, we are going to end up miserable. Shakespeare knew that. We need to remember it, and apply it in our lives.

8. *Inconsistency and too much "leeway"*

There is a trend towards treating the client as "consumer" rather than "patient". While I enthusiastically agree with this, I have learned it needs to be balanced by caution. As my clients keep reminding me, many (not all) addicts will get away with as much as possible while actively using. I have learned not to underestimate an addict's ingenuity to get past the "system".

Clients who are serious about staying clean will resent seeing others get away with cheating, and the program can lose credibility.

For example, a few years ago clinics started to "warn" clients the day before they were asked to give a urine sample, and staff no longer routinely supervised them. Although for many clients I would wish for them this less embarrassing practice, I believe this was a financial, not a clinical decision. In other words, for clients who want to cheat, this makes it way too easy.

Even closely supervised, too many clients know how to

give "bogus" urines (someone else's, or their own saved clean urine) As mentioned in a previous chapter, I will not go into details here, but suffice it to say, "never underestimate the active drug addict's ingenuity."

Some clinics now use the "swabs", which are much less intrusive than urines. There may be some evidence to support the idea that swabs are not as reliable as urine screens. Our clinic tried them, until some clients convinced our staff that they had gotten "false positives" for cocaine with swabs, (and, yes, that is possible). Word got out, and every client who had a swab positive for cocaine made the case that it was a false positive. We went back to using urine screens. Hopefully the technology will catch up, since the swabs are so much less humiliating than supervised urines. And, I fear unsupervised urines are just not very reliable.

It takes strong administration to set clear rules and not end up with clients feeling they are being treated like children. My first director continually quoted the phrase, *"no good deed remains unpunished."* It took me a few years at the clinic to really understand this: If you try to do one client a favor by letting a rule slide, shortly after that you will realize that every client has heard about it, and will expect to be treated that way.

9. *"A higher level of care": the little white lie*

When a client is unable to make progress on the clinic, and comes in seriously impaired day after day, misses doses, is noncompliant with treatment, or seems to be a danger to themselves or threatening to other clients or staff, we say they are inappropriate for the clinic, and need "a higher level of care." This is all true enough. But it is one of those convenient lies that we use to save face, and to feel better about the clients we can't help. The truth is usually that the "higher level of care" is unavailable to that client. It is easy to recommend, but often impossible to find, and if the client is not ready to get themselves admitted, there is no way to coerce them, unless they express suicidal or homicidal threats. If they do, we or their family can "section them" to a locked facility, and a week later they are back at our door, often still self destructive, and angrier than before..

This is a place where the system falls short. Often a client is smoking crack all day for weeks, not sleeping, and not eating. We know how risky their behavior is; they may be risking the chronic infections and other STDs, from sharing needles, paraphernalia, and often engaging in prostitution or other unsafe sex. They have no clue what they may be injecting into their veins, and they daily risk overdose or poisoning. I don't know what conclusion you would draw, but to me this person is a clear danger to themselves.

In our courts, however, it is often impossible to convince a judge that such a person needs to be kept safe for a few days until they can start thinking for themselves without the drug running their brain. There still seems to be a belief among many police and judges that if it is cocaine, (and remember the general belief is that cocaine is not "physically addicting"), then the person can just stop using. Even if that person is pregnant, we cannot protect the fetus. Even if the person is at the point at which they want to get "locked up" for a few days to detox, if their drug of choice is cocaine, we cannot get them admitted (see Chapter 1, #6).

Even when we get the client into a program, they usually know how to get out the next day if they choose. Sometimes they get kicked out even if they want to stay. Women who have survived their whole lives being fighters get kicked out because they fight with the other women. I once worked several days to get a man into a psychiatric ward because he was telling me that he had hidden an overdose ready to take if the voices in his head got any worse. The next day the psychiatrist threw him back out because he refused to attend groups. Something is wrong with that picture.

I absolutely agree that we cannot pay to have drug addicts do a "spin dry" in a detox every time they want to, and then go out immediately to get high again. But we need to come up with a way to help people stay safe when they are con- sciously or unconsciously destroying themselves. I know we need to protect the person's rights, but when the drug has control, there must be a way we can respectfully offer to contain the person in a safe place for an agreed time. And make sure they are going back to a safe place.

CHAPTER FOUR

What Works in Methadone Treatment

1. Respect: Using new ideas that work-

Harm reduction, Motivational Interviewing, & Cognitive Behavioral Therapy

When I started working in 1996, and for many years after that, our clinical staff was divided between two major methods of treating recovery: These were "abstinence" vs. "harm reduction models" of addiction treatment.

The **abstinence model** holds that addicts must be clean of all drugs or they will be refused further treatment. A relapse meant individuals lost what "clean time" they had accumulated. They were considered back "at square one" if they relapsed even briefly. There was a lot of confrontation, accusing the client of being in denial.

The **harm reduction model** is more forgiving. It's not that we don't encourage abstinence, but we might not worry about someone still smoking pot until they get the crack cocaine under control. We also will see improvement if someone is smoking crack twice a week when they had been using it daily. Someone who relapses but then gets right back on track is doing better than someone who has been using daily for years.

In this scenario, we acknowledge that improvement is better than nothing. We offer bleach kits (and sometimes clean syringes where those are not available) so that if the person is still shooting drugs, at least they cut down the chances of getting HIV or Hepatitis C (or spreading it). We offer condoms because, if they are prostituting, they are capable of keeping themselves somewhat safer.

The "harm reduction model" addiction treatment now concentrates on **"motivational interviewing."** This model accepts that the desire to change cannot be imposed on the client, but can only be nurtured and encouraged by staff. We now understand that addiction is a chronic condition, and relapse is to be learned from, not used to shame the user.

My job is to try to help people change their behavior. The old idea of confrontation often turns the client away from change.

Let me ask you again, dear reader, a personal question: When someone points their finger in your face and says, "You'd better do what I say!" does that motivate you to do what he or she tells you to do or not? Most likely you want to throw something at the person.

The concept of motivational interviewing is to respect where people are in their recovery, and try to encourage them to move towards health.

Cognitive Behavioral Therapy is a well respected method to promote change. This helps the addicted person (or anyone else) to identify some of their long held beliefs about themselves and the world that may not be true or helpful, and to understand that their behavior is driven by what they believe. It also teaches that their self destructive beliefs can be changed, and therefore the persons' lifelong destructive behaviors can change.

Those who believe that **"It's hopeless---nothing I do will help,"** will be less likely to even attempt new ways to improve their lives.

If they believe there is no way to calm a panic attack except to swallow a handful of benzos, then nothing a counselor says is going to deter them from that behavior next time they have a panic attack. The therapist has to first open the client's mind to the fact that maybe there are other ways to take back control of their own bodies, and then teach them those ways. This is not as easy as taking pills, but it does work, and it actually does more to improve the client's life. Clients who feel they can at least lessen or shorten that panic attack may begin to believe: "I can change this."

The same method can work for changing depression, anger, and any other uncomfortable emotions. And it is usually those uncomfortable emotions that trigger relapses.

Besides the appropriate medications, there are wonderful treatments for these symptoms. One problem I see is that people (not only people with addiction problems) really think there should be a pill to fix what they have been taught is a "chemical imbalance."

What I try to teach people is that the "chemical imbalance" is created by the beliefs they have about the world, themselves, and life. Each belief or thought drives the chemical production in their

brain. This can be changed by changing their way of thinking.

This is the basic "Cognitive Behavioral Theory." Our thoughts and beliefs drive our behavior. And while *I'm not saying it is easy*, these beliefs and thoughts can be changed. Someone who believes "nothing I do will help," might be able to change that to "I have more of a chance if I give something a try, even if I don't fully believe it can help." If they are able to at least try some new behaviors, then maybe one will work, and the person will be able to believe "maybe something I do will help."

This is not quite the same as the "affirmations" intervention used by many therapists. If I tell someone with terrible disgust of their own body to look in the mirror and repeat: "I am beautiful," most will ignore the instruction and think the therapist is incompetent. Clients need to identify thoughts that they can feel okay about saying to themselves. Maybe they can start with, "My eyes are okay."Positive thinking is very important, but it may have to be encouraged in small steps.

2. *Getting people into treatment more quickly*

This is a new idea, and I'm all for it, though I know it is a major headache for the staff members that have to make it work.

When someone has been living on the street and finally makes that decision to enter treatment, the very complex intake and titration process can be overwhelming. It can take a week or more even if the person is able to get to each appointment on time. The chaos of the street life, and still having to continue using to avoid withdrawal, makes this so difficult that the person often gets frustrated and gives up before getting their first dose.

Methadone is the most controlled prescribed drug in our country. Some of the red tape is being trimmed to allow people to get to dosing before all the paperwork is done, and this is a welcome relief. After they get dosed (titrated) it is easier for them to show up for appointments, and their heads are a lot clearer to answer questions and fill out the paperwork.

Our clinic has experimented with trying to do this once a week. They have all the required staff lined up for the process (urine screen, billing, physical, and titration) so they can dose the clients that day, if all goes well. However, if the intake urine they give has illicit methadone or benzos in it, this can disrupt the process. And this raises a question. A client might ask, "Why do I have to go use heroin when I can buy illicit methadone on the street and feel safer? It's a complicated issue. Another gray area: "Where do you draw the line?"

And then we need to find them counselors who have time to see them. As I said before, the idea that we try and keep clients for the money doesn't hold up to the reality test. There are plenty of clients coming into treatment. One concern I have is sometimes on those "quick intake" days our waiting room looks like a high school class- there are far too many young people who have become addicted to the pain pills.

3. *Supervised, reliable drug tests*

Even people who are strongly motivated to stay clean can be tempted if they are offered the drug and they think they will not be caught. Addiction is like a broken bone. The clinic with its rules, safety measures, and tests is like a cast meant to hold the bone in place until it can heal. It takes time and a lot of care.

I know some of my clients, who have plenty of clean time according to our records, have admitted to brief relapses which were not caught by the tests. And occasionally I receive reports of how some are still engaging in old risky behaviors---whether they are actually doing the drugs themselves, or making a connection for someone to get paid on the side. I know some have saved some portion of their take-homes and either sold it or helped out a friend. I realize there is a lot that goes on that I never hear about.

I know women who have been in prison seem to have a lot more knowledge regarding how to give "bogus" urines and get away with it. They pass on their legacy of knowledge. I'm still trying to figure out how one client, who was reported to be smoking crack daily, got through three supervised urines a week for about three months at DSS.

I have been fooled plenty of times.

If I hear about cheating the tests to this degree, the clients hear a lot more. The more they hear about people "getting over" on the clinic, the more that old addictive voice whispers in their heads, "Why should I try to stay clean and do things right if others are getting away with it?"

I am hoping that the swabs will become more widely accepted and reliable (and affordable). But there are plenty of reports by clients that they have ways to cheat on those too.

Reliable, well supervised drug screenings are essential.

4. *Clear rules, with plenty of second chances*

I guess the trick is to have a heavy enough "hammer" to help clients resist the temptations, but not so heavy that they give up in discouragement.

The other important piece is the balance between consistent rules for all clients, with enough room to take individual circumstances into consideration.

When someone is using cocaine and has no support system to help them stop (and remember, there are few programs and no inpatient detox for cocaine), it takes a lot to balance the all-consuming effect of that drug.

Sometimes I will be working with a client who is about to be detoxed ("thrown off") the clinic for non-compliance (consistent cocaine urines). We can mandate them to lots of groups, but at the end of the day those people (even if they are really trying to stay clean) will be going home to that same chaotic environment, where they walk past the drug dealer on the way home, or have to go by a crack addict's open door where they can smell the drug in the air, or they can get home only to have a brother, or cousin, or friend, arrive with the drug, wanting someplace to shoot up or smoke it, and offer a share.

Even if a person slips up and uses, if they are using only two times a week instead of daily, then that is progress. And the urines will remain "dirty" and won't show that progress. So sometimes you need to take the small gains, and acknowledge that the person is trying. And yes, sometimes they "get over on you."

Some clients will go through every appeal, and actually be put on a detox before they find the strength to put down that drug. I have seen this happen, and at that very last chance they pull themselves back. But sometimes they don't.

For young people with good immune systems, a detox is extremely unpleasant but they can get through it. But for some, who have already done a lot of damage to themselves, a fast detox can be very risky. And, of course, few people get through a detox without going back to street drugs until they can get back on the clinic. This puts them at risk for overdose, harmful "cuts" in the drug, and of course illegal activity which can put them into more danger of violence and set them back with new criminal charges.

I am reminded of what I learned back in 1973 when I was working in a program for "emotionally disturbed adolescents." There are kids who, if you "give them an inch" will definitely take the proverbial "mile". They will see your good intentions as weakness, and try to take you for all they can get. Then there are the others, who are so used to being slapped down every time they slip... These kids are so surprised and grateful when someone cuts them a little slack and tries to help them instead of punishing them that they will try very hard to deserve the chance. I see people caught in addictive behaviors fall into the same categories.

My belief is that a good counselor will try to distinguish between these, without letting their ego get "taken in" by the more "personable" clients. I would rather make a mistake in trying to give someone the benefit of the doubt (at least once) even if it means I am sometimes seen as naive, or easy to "get over on"

I try to remain just skeptical enough to take all stories with a "grain of salt", strong enough not to take lies and manipulation personally, and patient enough to see the desperation just behind the bravado.

5. *Strong rewards for any progress*

Take-homes are the most obvious reward when people are on the clinic. Methadone, as the most controlled pharmaceutical in the country, must be dispensed daily by the medical staff.

This means that clients are extremely restricted in their movements. Skipping a dose means feeling sick by morning for most (some say they can skip one without feeling the effects). If the individuals work early in the morning, they have to get to the clinic before they are supposed to be at work. Often they are met at the clinic with news that they must give a urine test that morning, or see their counselor or the medical staff. This adds stress to their work day, and often (depending on the job) makes work impossible for the time being.

In our city, fishing is one of the main industries, and fishermen are usually unable to get on the clinic because they cannot go on the trips overnight. *(Suboxone has been a help to those fisherman that want to take their recovery seriously, but unfortunately it is more often used only il- licitly until they get off the boat with their money, and are met on the docks by the dealers.)*

For others, spontaneous overnight trips (vacations or family visits) become problematic. These must be planned weeks in advance, setting up "courtesy dosing" at other clinics. This is where the clients get the idea that "methadone is liquid handcuffs."

So the idea of getting the first take-home dose is usually a milestone. At our clinic the client can apply 45 days after the first clean urine screen (if a few other requirements are met). As soon as clients have earned one take-home, they are allowed to take more on special occasions that can be documented, so travel is easier.

More take-homes are added over the months to follow, until after eighteen months of being clean, clients only have to come to the clinic once a week. After another six months they can come once every two weeks. This is great for allowing clients to have a "life" beyond the clinic.

Other rewards are hard to arrange. I believe some clinics are able to reward successful clients by giving them more control of policies through a **client advisory board**. Our clinic has a very troubled history of such attempts. Attempts have been undermined by power struggles---the attempt by someone the other clients do not respect to take too much control, or the rumors that the CAB members are "rats" in cahoots with the administration, and so are despised by other clients. I still hope to see a successful CAB happen at some point.

I know one of the difficulties is that clients who would be the most effective are often reluctant to have their association with the clinic made more public. It's a difficult problem.

A successful client advisory board needs to feel they have some actual access to at least being heard by the administration. I believe it is important that clients be able to give some feedback on policy changes before these are enacted. Methadone clients are often feeling very powerless about having any control over their own lives. A successful CAB can be very empowering.

6. *On-site psychiatric help*

Mental health needs to be addressed in coordination with substance abuse treatment. Most addicts were pulled into their addictions by mental health problems, whether anxiety, social phobia, obsessive compulsive disorder, depression, or post traumatic stress disorder. And if they did not have the diagnosis when they got into substance abuse, the drug world most likely has given them their share of trauma by the time they reach treatment.

Sometimes addictive behaviors are tied in to the clients' role in their family. When possible and appropriate, family therapy can be an important part of treatment. Learning social skills, when someone grew up never having constructive social models, can be essential.

Communication between the counselor and the psychiatrist is ideal. If someone sees a psychiatrist outside the clinic, there is often little communication. I have found that some clients try to keep their psychiatrist from even knowing that they are on the clinic. While I understand that the client does not want the "stigma" of methadone to affect his relationship with his doctor, this can be dangerous, especially if the doctor is prescribing benzodiazepines or other narcotic drugs.

Clients involved in substance abuse have usually chosen their psychiatrist on the advice of others "on the street", and these physicians are often the ones that can be counted on to write the scripts that the clients want.

I feel the daily interaction between counselors and the prescribers is extremely helpful. Clients are often very good at appearing alert at their psychiatrist's office, and then they nod off at counseling or group. They may not have a relationship with the prescriber and may say everything is fine when they are having difficulties or "playing doctor" themselves, not taking some meds or not taking them as prescribed.

The counselors can also report to the prescribers if they notice significant changes in their clients. I appreciate having input to giving a client a diagnosis, since I am allowed more time to get to know the client.

I know that on-site psychiatric help is rare at a methadone clinic. But I believe it is an important piece of treatment.

7. *Inpatient detox for cocaine, more effective long term residential programs, and "Safe Houses"*

As discussed earlier, the transition between residential programs and methadone clinic still comprises a serious gap in our drug treatment system. Many (not all) of my more successful clients have come through a long residential program.

Clients have called me in desperation because they've just been terminated (maybe deservedly, maybe not) from a program they'd been in for months. Having been dropped off, late on a Friday, they had little chance of staying clean, since transfer back to a methadone clinic had not been already arranged. By Monday morning they were well into a relapse, and still feeling sick.

Even if they are back on the methadone clinic when they get out, if they can't get into a sober house quickly, they are most likely to go back to the places they know best. It will be nearly impossible for them to remain clean if the only place they can go is with friends from the crack house.

Since most sober houses are privately run they can be very good, or they can be very bad. I often hear that drugs are readily available within many of these programs.

To fix the system we need more consistency and some streamlining between detoxes, residential programs and sober houses. If this is not taken over by government (and yes, I know that is more tax dollars and more red tape) then we need some kind of oversight.

8. Group process

I am not going to argue for or against AA and NA or other 12-step programs. The statistics show that this works for many people. Many of my clients put their faith in these programs, and feel it has saved their lives.

I will not say that it works for everyone, because many of my clients have gone that route and failed, and they are grateful to find alternatives that allow a new way to work on their recovery.

Some of my most successful clients, who have gotten off methadone and stayed clean for several years (so far so good...), have not wanted to be involved with these programs.

Often it is because they feel unwelcome and shamed by the reputation of methadone treatment. Some attend anyway, but choose to not say anything about being on the clinic, but that puts them in a position of lying right from the start, which goes against everything being taught.

Some are agnostic and can't relate to the idea of "a higher power." Yes, you are supposed to be able to use other ideas besides God as your higher power, but most meetings and related literature are very much God-centered. This is wonderful if you are comfortable with that. Not so good if you aren't. I do want people to go to meetings if they feel it helps them, but I want them to know that recovery can happen in other ways.

The best known alternative is "Rational Recovery." It is basically a cognitive behavioral therapy model and goes by many other names. There are plenty of good websites available.

I was fortunate to attend a graduate program that believed in group process. Groups can help anyone, if they are supportive, and help people to feel they are not alone. Clients must be convinced that they can have a safe place to talk, and are encouraged to work on the problems that face them. This goes for cancer as well as for drug recovery. We are social animals and need to feel connected to others.

There are a very few clients who have such overwhelming problems in social settings, either from anxiety or rage, that they are not appropriate to attend groups. Some clients are not trusted in a group. The group can quickly fall apart around such a client. Clients who repeatedly show up impaired, or "nod off" can detract from others' experience or trigger drug cravings.

But group experience can be what helps clients realize that they are not alone, that others have felt what they feel, and that others have turned their lives around and maybe they can do it too.

Groups provide the best opportunity for clients to get feedback about how they are acting, and it shows the counselor a much clearer picture of the interpersonal problems the client needs to work on.

9. *Encouraging clients who are stable to slowly detox--without deadlines-*

Remember that though the goal is to have a client get off methadone if possible, there is a lot of work the client needs to do before they attempt it.

For the family and others who want to see the client off the clinic:

We all would like to see clients able to put opiate addiction behind them. We wish they could get through the physical symptoms and *ta-da*, they would be done with it. , and they and you could get on with life.

I hate to tell you this, but it is not going to be that easy.

First, you need to know that even the best intentioned family member might be doing something which is either enabling or impeding progress for the addicted loved one. Try to examine your own part of the pattern. If you are enabling, get some help to figure out how to step back in a healthy way. Try to find support for yourself, and if what you have been doing isn't helping, see if there is a different way to look at the situation. **If you are ashamed that someone in your family is on methadone, realize that is "your stuff" and that pushing this person to hurry off methadone might just be making the problem worse.**

For the methadone client:

Remember:
    the slower the better
    the lower the dose, the slower it has to be

Listen to what your body is telling you. Don't try to "tough it out." Don't keep pushing the detox if you start feeling sick---you are likely to get yourself deep into withdrawal by the time you admit it, and you'll have to go up on your dose higher than before in order to stabilize.

If you can keep the detox slow and steady, you will have a much better chance to succeed. During that time, use your counseling and support groups to figure out the reasons you ended up with this problem. Use the time to get into safe surroundings, and set up a plan regarding where you want to go next with your life.

It can be done, but there are worse things than staying on the clinic.

10. *Help with reintegrating into the community*

This is a tough one. There is a deep prejudice against "junkies."

This may have to start within the recovery community. You may have to rely on some very brave people saying, "Hey, I was on methadone and it helped me." We hear a lot about the celebrities fighting addiction, but it is usually part of a scandal or because they overdose.

People are not likely to talk about their experience on methadone if, as a result, they may lose their job, or have their family threaten them with banishment, or have an ex-spouse threaten that they will lose custody of their kids.

Families could help by encouraging their loved one to continue in a treatment that is working for them. Maybe people who call themselves "Christians" can try to take the advice that Jesus told the crowd who wanted to stone the woman caught in adultery: "He who has never sinned, throw the first stone." To me that is the cornerstone of Christianity, but I rarely hear it preached.

Maybe if a friend or someone in your family has been helped by methadone, you could speak up and say that. Maybe if you are an employer and an applicant comes up positive for methadone you could talk to them, make sure it is legal, but don't automatically rule out that person as an employee.

I was so proud of one client a few years ago who was back in college. She was in a psychology class doing a chapter on addictions. The professor brought in an "expert." The guest speaker started to skim over methadone treatment with all the normal scorn, derision and eye-rolling, implying "we all know that doesn't work," and my client (who had just been struggling with panic attacks whenever she had to do any public speaking) gathered her strength (and this woman has considerable strength) spoke up and said, "It worked for me."

I think that is what it will take.

11. *Opportunities and incentives to get off disability and earn a decent wage*

One of the most despised things about the stereotypical methadone client is that they are often on social security disability.

I would argue that, at first, this is the only option for many. Their lives are usually in absolute chaos when they begin treatment, and they have pretty much burned every bridge available to them. Family and friends are not about to trust them in their homes after giving them too many chances. Sometimes the families are not even safe for the client--- some of my clients are third generation heroin addicts.

They need to get a steady enough income to get out of the crack house and have a safe place to work on their recovery. They need health insurance to get them into treatment.

But let's say they have that, and they are feeling ready to try to get a job or get back to school.
Remember that, for most clients, disability income is going to provide only a poverty-level lifestyle. (And yes, there are those who are scamming and seem to do just fine, but I'm talking about the ones who want to do things right.)

I recall one client who had come from the street. She was raised in a drug-addicted family, and had been a prostitute. She'd been in jail, and had recently graduated from the local "Drug Court" program. Despite all this, she was very personable, and had a positive attitude. She got into CNA classes, studied hard, and graduated with great grades.

She loved her grandmother, who was in a local nursing home. My client had been a frequent visitor there for years. She was liked by the other residents and the staff. When they heard she was graduating, they gave her a job. As part of the process they did a background check, and after two weeks of working (and loving it), the CORI came back, and she came in devastated. They had to fire her.

Now, I understand that elderly people have to be protected and I understand this wasn't the methadone (which is legal and confidential) that kept her from working, but it is typical of the lifestyle. Criminal histories can prevent people from job offerings---people who would probably do great at a job. And they end up back on public money, or back in illegal activity which will pass them back into the legal system. Another vicious cycle.

I know there are people all over our country who have been able to get back into work after methadone treatment, sometimes, while they still were in treatment, without the employers finding out. This is becoming more difficult as more employers are testing not only for illegal drugs, but for methadone. Legally the employer cannot fire someone because they are on methadone, but they can most likely find some legal reason not to hire them,

It is scary for someone to let go of that disability check. Social Security has improved this some, but people still trade horror stories and they are scared.

To make our system work better we will need to find better ways to help people earn a decent living after drug treatment, including methadone (or Suboxone) treatment. Either that, or we must reconcile ourselves to the fact that we will have to continue to support many of them through public funds.

One of the very hopeful programs currently helping people who would otherwise have little hope of getting past their drug abuse and criminal history was reported on 60 Minutes. It showed people learning skills and earning a decent living at D.C. Central Kitchen, with the help of Chef Jose Andres. The program hires the disadvantaged, teaches them culinary arts, uses donated surplus food, and feeds the homeless. Let's initiate some more programs along these lines.

CHAPTER FIVE

Some Hard Decisions

1. *"the Reality Principle"*

Something I learned years ago at a conference about education reform seems very relevant here:

It is the "reality principle": **Is what you are doing getting you what you want?**

When we are trying to get someone to change their behavior, (stop using illicit drugs) and we are frustrated by the results, then we need to evaluate whether what we are doing is getting us the desired result. Everything we do needs to be put through that "filter."

Otherwise another saying comes into play---the popular definition of insanity: **"Insanity is doing the same thing over and over and expecting different results."**

There are some things that we are doing right in opiate drug treatment, but there is also much that does not work. Let's try to figure out what works, and what doesn't.

2. *Disability/methadone- A formula for depression and obesity*

Let's consider- What "should be" and what "is."

As I was attending college in the late sixties and early seventies, my "hippie" liberal views were a bone of contention between me and my staunch Republican father. As most young people do, I followed my heart and felt we, the educated and economically comfortable, could fix poverty by offering financial support to the poor. Don't get me wrong, I still believe we need to help solve these problems which are even more alarming today. But I also see that some of the solutions are not as simple as they seemed. I am working with a population in which many are third generation welfare/disability recipients, and I see how a "given" income (though necessary for a few), becomes a trap for the many.

I see the damage done by well meaning programs, and though I support an individual's rights, I see many gray areas. **I see how necessary the disability program is, and I also see too much fraud, and too many checks going to the drug dealers**. We need some accountability built into these programs, and people accepting disability checks need some way to feel they are earning their keep.

I have seen the e-mail going around (several times over the past few years) sometimes called "Urine or You're out" and appreciate and sympathize with the anger. It is difficult to understand why we who pay taxes out of hard earned income might have to submit to urine tests to keep our jobs. Yet somehow it comprises a violation of human rights to ask someone on public assistance/disability to take a drug test. There must be a way to respectfully do this. Otherwise it's a system that enables addiction.

And the health risks multiply as people who tend to be depressed anyway have no need to get up in the morning and no incentive to try and work on the problems that have caused the disability.

One of the sad scenarios I see is young people coming on the clinic, getting on disability (often because their parents are on it), and embracing the belief that they now are set for life. They are condemning themselves to a life in poverty, or of scamming to survive comfortably.

This is not to take away from those who do need the disability payments and try to do the right thing with them. The system is needed, but we have every reason to try and make it work more efficiently.

Everyone needs a purpose in life. If we let people crippled by addiction and mental illness be labeled, or learn to label themselves as permanently disabled, we are setting them up for depression and relapse.

3. *Rethinking Pain treatment-*

We, individually, and as a culture, have to rethink how to treat, and how to deal with chronic pain.

As described in Chapter 3, some have grown up seeing their adult caregivers hiding their pain with alcohol or prescription medications, or they were taught that they should not have to feel discomfort, or they learned that discomfort is something terrible and that they must rely on something outside themselves to help them feel better. Without doubt, these people will grow up to have a difficult time getting through the ups and downs of life without turning to their drug of choice for comfort.

This cultural change will mean educating doctors to help

clients understand the limitations of pain management. It will mean educating patients that they have a role in their pain management. If they have gained significant weight, that should be part of the focus of treatment. To help alleviate the pain in their knees, the person needs to work on diet and exercise before surgery or opiates. If neuropathy has to do with type 2 diabetes, then diet should be addressed. If someone with breathing problems is still smoking cigarettes, then cessation needs to be the focus before asking the government or the insurance to pay huge sums on breathing treatments. If lifestyle changes can improve fibromyalgia symptoms, then that needs to be addressed.

But let us try to make this supportive, not punitive. Remember, shaming people does not help get us the result we want.

When opiates are used in treatment, patients should be educated on the problem of withdrawal.

I have a dear friend who went through radiation for throat cancer. He was put on Roxicet (liquid Percocet) for over a year. One day he mentioned that his legs were aching terribly, that he was waking up sweating, and having difficulty sleeping. Then he mentioned that he had just gone off his Roxicet. His doctor (a well respected cancer doctor), had not even thought to mention that he would go through withdrawal when it was discontinued.

Doctors are now allowed to give methadone pills for pain, though they are not supposed to give them for "methadone maintenance" (for addiction). Of course there are the clients who have a history of addiction who also have legitimate chronic pain issues. That seems like a very "gray area" to me.

Some doctors are fine with giving the pills indefinitely for chronic pain. However, without the structure of the clinic, this means that the patient doesn't usually have to submit to routine urine screens or blood levels. That is fine for the client dedicated to not abusing the pills, but it would take a very savvy doctor to distinguish those capable of handling this treatment and those who aren't. I would even bet that the doctor who thinks he can distinguish between them will be fooled. As stated, most recent "methadone deaths" are not typically clients at a methadone clinic, but at a pain clinic.

We, as a culture, need to look at how we think of, and how we treat chronic pain issues. When I bring this up, many clients (at the clinic, but also in my private practice) think I am saying that their pain is not "real." We need to educate our clients that pain can be very real and still be helped with lifestyle intervention and cognitive behavioral therapy (CBT).

While opiates are extremely effective in acute, short term pain management, they are limited in effectiveness, just as heroin is, by the way our bodies adjust and increase our tolerance for opiates. We now know that chronic pain often improves with changes we, as patients, can control---that is, by losing weight, quitting smoking, getting more exercise....

Some studies are showing that CBT actually works better (and lasts longer) than pills do for chronic pain.

I encourage anyone interested in this to check out the "Medscape" website (it is free but you need to register) and type in "CBT" to search. Studies are indicating that CBT is better than pills for many ailments, including insomnia and lower back pain, and better in conjunction with meds than meds alone for depression and anxiety.

Pain is a part of life, and we all need to learn that pills can only do so much. The part of treatment that we often don't want to hear about is that we have to do a lot of the work ourselves to manage our pain.

As the serenity prayer says, there are things we can change, and other things we just have to accept (or spend our life feeling miserable about.).

4. *Rethinking Anxiety treatment-*

Just about anyone who goes to their primary care physician and says they are suffering from panic attacks is likely to walk out with a prescription for benzodiazepines.

Many people today suffer constant overwhelming anxiety, often with panic attacks. These symptoms limit their lives, some so acutely that they cannot work. I can't tell you how many people I see (addicts and non-addicts) who say going to the grocery store is a huge ordeal because of panic attacks.

Many people have good reason to feel that the world is not a safe place, and that whatever they do, they cannot keep themselves safe. I can understand why they feel they want to give up and hide behind the blissful "forgetfulness" of benzodiazepines (there are also alternatives like SOMA, a muscle relaxant and some over-the-counter meds that can have similar effects).

I would wish that benzodiazepines were as closely watched as methadone is, with much better education for physicians prescribing them.

As with pain, we have been led to believe that anxiety is something we need to fix with a pill.

This is another thing we need to rethink. People with chronic anxiety need to know there are better options to control their symptoms rather than only numbing them with medication. When the pill wears off, the problems are still there. Often they are worse because people have been sleeping too much, or were too "foggy" from the medication to deal with the problems. They have often neglected daily chores- the dishes and laundry have not gotten themselves done; the abusive partner may still be there. And so the person takes another pill.

If you are actually in danger, it is not "clinical anxiety", but fear. Fear is our body's way of telling us to do something to get out of danger.

If the anxiety is from a current unsafe situation, such as domestic violence, then taking the pills will only prolong the problem.

If the anxiety is from the past, as it is with people who grew up in abusive homes, or who have suffered a catastrophic accident that took away their belief of safety in the world, then therapy can help. We now have very effective treatments for anxiety and panic. Pills only fuzz out the anxiety but do nothing to change it. When the person stops taking the pill, the fears are there waiting, more overwhelming than ever. When people who lose a loved one want to avoid the terrible feelings of loss, they can take these pills. When they have to stop the pills, the grief feelings are still there, fresh as a new wound, waiting to be processed. Grief must be faced and worked through.

If the anxiety is chronic the person may have never known what their body feels like to be relaxed and feel safe. The new "mindfulness" techniques work if they are learned and practiced. (Too many people try it a few times and decide "I can't do it"-it takes self discipline)

I have seen clients who were sure they couldn't survive without their pills, but they were forced off them (slowly detoxed) by a doctor. And I have seen these people come alive, and do much better facing life as it is, instead of hiding from it.

I think often we don't give ourselves enough credit. We can deal with a lot more than we think we can.

Anxiety is also a part of life. Pills can only do so much. We need to work at helping ourselves. We need to take care of the problems causing the anxiety, and do our own personal work at trying to find some meaning to life. A pill won't do that for us.

5. *More comprehensive (and realistic) treatment for cocaine*

Let's revisit the actual cost of not having a way to keep people safe from themselves when they are caught up in cocaine use. The money saved by not covering a detox might be small compared with the actual cost of the illegal activity, disability fraud, welfare and children's services.

The hope of a pill to help "block" the high of cocaine is not looking good in studies. However, there was a report on a vaccine which seemed to show some signs of success (found on the NIDA website)

Unless there is a "silver bullet" found very soon, then let's find a way in which people can "sign themselves in" to a long enough program to let them reclaim their brains from the overwhelming power this drug has over the addicted person.

6. *The rights of the unborn child vs. the rights of the addicted mother*

An aside for those wondering about the effect of methadone on pregnancy: Although it does have complications, methadone is a much safer alternative to illegal drugs. The methadone is longer acting, so the fetus is not put through constant extremes of highs and withdrawal symptoms that it would go through with street opiates. Anyone trying to tell a pregnant woman to get off of methadone is risking her relapse-and increasing the danger of miscarriage or premature birth. If she is feeling withdrawal, then the baby is feeling withdrawal. Pregnant women are the only clients who are allowed to be escorted from jail to get their dose, for the baby's sake. The clinic cannot detox a pregnant woman from methadone.

How can we, as a society, protect the unborn child whose mother is smoking crack, or using other illicit drugs, throughout the pregnancy?

This is a very explosive, difficult area. I know it is "politically incorrect" to propose any legally mandated intervention.

And, yes, it is a 'slippery slope". It is also something that needs to be discussed in a way that is respectful both to the addicted woman and to her unborn child.

Some states have passed laws mandating that if a woman who is pregnant is found to be actively using illicit drugs, she will be given the choice to have an abortion or go in-patient until she gives birth. These laws are being found to violate the rights of the woman, and are being overturned. I agree that these laws are punitive, and do not take into account the complexities of the addiction.

Upon searching this subject on the web, I discovered a lot of discussion regarding whether the woman should be charged as a criminal after the birth, and tried for abuse and neglect. This seems to miss the most important point; we already know that criminalizing the addict does little to prevent the behavior. Meanwhile, we know that such action would mean more women would avoid any prenatal care, increasing harm to the infants.

Some of the blogs about this problem focus, instead, on making sure the women are offered treatment. Of course. We want to believe that a woman in that situation would gladly and of her own free will, accept the help for the good of her child. Many would. Many do. But, I have seen women becoming pregnant again, though they have already lost at least one child to DSS. Others continue prostituting while pregnant, are homeless, and are using illegal drugs. These are women who already have treatment available. I know of one woman who has lost six children to Social Services.

Something more is needed.

One of my clients has a sister who was pregnant and using cocaine. He and I commiserated that, until birth, the baby had no rights, yet the minute it was born the state would take custody. And, although there are many couples who would love to adopt an infant, these infants already have many strikes against them.

RJ's law- A young man, who has many serious disabilities due (most likely) to his mother's use of drugs during her pregnancy, drew up a law that was designed to protect these children. It was also overturned. Please look this one up online (just do a search for "RJ's law.") It is heartbreaking, and I know I was one of many appalled that we cannot protect these kids.

I can also see the "slippery slope" part- Where do we stop? Clearly, cigarettes also put a baby at risk. I would suggest that we should, at least, deal with the effects of illegal drugs. Cigarettes are still legal. Cocaine and methamphetamine are not. Maybe we need to draw the line somewhere.

Unfortunately, in view of the public's disdain for a drug-using pregnant woman, any legal response is likely to be met with disgust and condemnation, and tend towards punishment, not support. Let's remember again that Christian teaching: "Judge not, that you be not judged" and "He who is without sin throw the first stone."

I have heard of one doctor who was able to show a pregnant woman the effect of the cocaine on her baby by having her watch a sonogram while she used. Apparently this was convincing enough to this woman to convince her to put herself in long term treatment.

While I can't imagine ethics allowing this anymore (having a pregnant woman using illegal drugs in a medical facility), maybe showing a video such as this one might persuade some women to protect themselves and their fetus. Maybe it could be shown to substance abuse clients of child bearing age in any program or in jails. Maybe it could be included in sex education in health classes. (I would hope this is being discussed in the places this is allowed) We could also show the effects of cigarettes on the fetus. (Studies are showing the possibility of ADHD being connected to prenatal exposure to cigarettes). Maybe, along with easier access to "amnesty," non-judgmental, supportive long term treatment programs would be enough to help reduce the number of children exposed.

It would be a start.

7. *Better support for dealing with Domestic Violence issues*

Shall I tell you how many women have confided that when they were pregnant their boyfriends have kicked them in the belly during fights?

SOME HARD DECISIONS

Have you seen the percentage of murders that are DV related?

And my experience in regard to police involvement is that the calls of a woman are not always taken seriously.

I understand that police grow frustrated trying to repeatedly help a woman, only to see her back walking with that same boyfriend a couple days later.

But this "vicious circle" is caused partly by the fact that when the woman finally summons the courage to call the police and actually follows through with taking out a restraining order, she is not confident that she will get a response quickly enough if she does call 911 the next time. It is just easier to go back to "the devil you know."

And I have seen the boyfriends get out after months of "continuances" with a "slap on the wrist" by judges that seem much too understanding of the abusive man's point of view.

We need more educational and supportive programs to change the very ingrained cultural acceptance of this chronic violence.

Just think of how many children might avoid the trap of addiction if they are not raised in constant terror.

CHAPTER SIX

The Future of Opiate Treatment-

The problem that won't go away

So, let's diagnose the state of opiate treatment as desperate, but not hopeless.

There are still alternative treatments being tried.

I believe it won't be a one treatment fits-all solution. It won't be either methadone, or Suboxone, or Narcan patches. It will be what works for each client. People usually do better with choices.

Opiate addiction is complex and devastating. As much as we'd all like a "quick fix", we are unlikely to find one.

I believe that methadone will have a place in treatment for a long time.

Remember that the worst thing about methadone is also the best thing. It is hard to get off of it. This means people will come for their dose, and the longer they stay in treatment, the more likely they are to put their lives back together

Of course there will be those clients who continue to abuse the "tool" of methadone, using the clinic only to ward off withdrawal; but there will also be many who desperately want to get help and to do it right.

Remember that there are clients who get off of methadone, but these aren't the ones you hear about, and they aren't the ones hanging around the clinic complaining about "liquid handcuffs".

These are the ones who quietly get their take-homes, pay off debts, clear up old legal issues, get more stable housing and safer friends, resolve their psychiatric issues, get back to school or vocational training, and slowly detox---though they will not advertise their success due to the stigma that accompanies methadone treatment.

For those that do not feel they can give up the structure of the clinic, they too can mend their lives, and keep the security of the methadone clinic for a fraction of the cost of the crimes they would be committing, or the price of keeping them in jail.

For those who think that once people have conquered the physical withdrawal of the opiate, an addict should be able to return to "normal" life, think of how many people get through the physical withdrawal from cigarettes (or chocolate, for that matter) and how many relapse.

One of the most destructive forces in methadone treatment is the disdain for it by the general public. As with all prejudices, it is easy to distrust and dislike anonymous groups; it is harder when you see a face, know their fears, and hear their stories.

I hope the future brings a wider acceptance of methadone. Let's take what we've got that works, and try to fix the parts that need fixing.

Education of the general public would help demystify heroin addiction, bring it out of the shadows, and allow it to be viewed as fundamentally the same as other harmful addictions. We must also understand methadone is an important treatment option. This may happen sooner rather than later, because so many young people are falling into opiate addiction through abusing prescription pain pills.

Success will depend on a more complete support system: first, inpatient for acute care, (including respite/detox for cocaine), safe housing options, and then a more effective way to help people get off of welfare/disability and into employment that offers some possibility of regaining dignity and of earning a comfortable wage. For those unable to work, I would love to see some requirement of time spent either in community service, or in treatment for that disability.

On a wider perspective:

Beyond the treatment itself, success is also tied to some larger cultural change. To make a lasting impact on addiction, we will have to confront some fundamental problems--- especially how we think about and treat mental health problems and handle anxiety and pain management.

We all need to remember, and to teach our children, that there isn't a pill that will fix all problems. There are some very uncomfortable feelings we just need to feel, and find out we can get through them. For some problems, we need to work on fixing the source, whether it is to eat healthier, or exercise, or give up an old familiar crutch, be it heroin, cigarettes, cookies, or crack.

Addiction can't be contained by jail, and it won't be ignored. It will continue to pull down our culture until we acknowledge its power and grapple with it in realistic and effective ways.

Bibliography

Cassels, Caroline. Medscape, Medical News, 2009. (www.medscape.com) **Medically Prescribed Heroin Superior to Methadone for Severe, Refractory Opioid dependence.**

Jeffrey, Susan. Medscape Medical News 2008: **Methadone Dosages Correlate Poorly with Serum Levels.**

Leavitt, Shinderman, Maxwell, Eap, & Paris: **When "Enough" is not Enough**: The Mount Sinai Journal of Medicine Vol. 67 Nos.5&6 October/November 2000.

Medscape, Medical News, 2008.(www.medscape.com) **Recovering Heroin Addicts Fare Better on Opiate Maintenance Therapy.**

Methadone myths and Facts: CAMH Center for Addiction and Mental Health (online)

New York: Drug Policy Alliance 2006 (online) **About Methadone & Buprenorphine**: Revised Second Edition.

NIDA (www.NIDA.nih.gov) (National Institute of Drug Abuse):**"Methadone at Forty."**

NIDA (www.NIDA.nih.gov) Notes Volume 22, Number2: **Methadone Reduces Rats' Cocaine Seeking.**

PLNDP and Join Together-(January 2000) **A Physician's Guide on How to Advocate for More Effective National and State Policies**. Quoted in National Council Magazine 2007, Volume 2.

SAMHSA: http://www.samhsa.gov

Schottenfeld,R.S., Chawarski,M.C. Pakes,J.R., Pantolon,M.V., Carroll,K.M. and Kosten,T.R. **Methadone versus Buprenorphine**, American Journal of Psychiatry; 162(2) 2005.

CPSIA information can be obtained at www.ICGtesting.com
Printed in the USA
LVOW12s0908231114

415189LV00004B/673/P